The Art of Telling Bad News Well

Dr. h.c. Jalid Sehouli, MD

Medical Director and Professor
Center of Oncological Surgery and
Department of Gynecology
Charité Comprehensive Cancer Center
Medical University of Berlin
Berlin, Germany

Translated by Noah Block-Harley

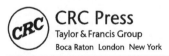

CRC Press
Taylor & Francis Group
Boca Raton London New York

CRC Press is an imprint of the
Taylor & Francis Group, an **informa** business

Originally authored in the German language by Jalid Sehouli with the original title *Von der Kunst, schlechte Nachrichten gut zu überbringen*; © 2018 by Kösel Verlag, a division of Verlagsgruppe Random House GmbH, München, Germany

CRC Press
Taylor & Francis Group
6000 Broken Sound Parkway NW, Suite 300
Boca Raton, FL 33487-2742

English language edition © 2020 by Taylor & Francis Group, LLC
CRC Press is an imprint of Taylor & Francis Group, an Informa business

No claim to original U.S. Government works

Printed on acid-free paper

Printed by CPI Group (UK) Ltd, Croydon CR0 4YY

International Standard Book Number-13: 978-0-367-35668-2 (Paperback)
978-0-367-36474-8 (Hardback)

Library of Congress Control Number: 2019947616

Visit the Taylor & Francis Web site at
http://www.taylorandfrancis.com

and the CRC Press Web site at
http://www.crcpress.com

Contents

Acknowledgments

Thanks to all those without whom this book would never have been possible. It began with a meeting, followed by conversation, experience, memory, and understanding. Then, and only then, came this book.

I would especially like to thank:

All the patients, relatives, friends, and colleagues who placed their trust in me; Dr. Elke Leonhard, Dr. Tobias Winstel, and Karin Stuhldreier for their tremendous support; and the whole team at Kösel Verlag—thanks to readers Hans Georg Hoffmann, Marlene Fritsch, and Noah Block-Harley. A special thanks to my colleague and partner in our Breaking Bad News seminars, Dr. Christine Klapp, and my mentor, Wolfgang Kohlhaase, and a thousand thanks to my terrific kids and my wonderful wife, Mrs. Adak Pirmorady.

Jalid Sehouli

Author

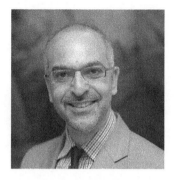

Professor Dr. med. h.c. Jalid Sehouli is a German gynecologist and oncologist who specializes in peritoneal and ovarian cancer. He is a professor at the famous Berlin's Charité Hospital and a writer of scientific as well as philosophic works.

Dr. Sehouli is the son of Moroccan parents who fled from Morocco in the 1960s and were illiterate. He grew up in the Berlin working-class district of Wedding. While training to become a nurse, he was offered a place to study medicine at the Free University of Berlin. He studied there from 1989 to 1995. In 1998, he earned his doctorate with a thesis on "Post-Operative Use of Unconventional Cancer Therapies in Gynecological Oncology." He was certified in 2002 as a specialist in gynecology and obstetrics.

In 2005, he was appointed to teach gynecology and obstetrics. Two years later, in 2007, he accepted the offer of a W2 professorship at Berlin's Charité Hospital. In 2014, he was selected for the W3 full professorship for Gynecology for life at the Charité and has since been director of the Clinic for Gynaecology and a full professor at the Charité and leads one of the largest and most famous gynecological cancer centers there.

Dr. Sehouli also specializes in experimental surgical gynecology and oncosurgery, as well as the subject of doctor–patient communication (e.g., breaking bad news). Dr. Sehouli is the coeditor of various professional journals and the author (first, senior, or coauthor) of several hundred articles in national and international journals on all aspects of gynecology with an emphasis on diagnosis, therapy, and aftercare in gynecological oncology. He has performed several international surveys about patients' preferences and patients' expectations.

In 2012, Dr. Sehouli published his first work of fiction and philosophy, *Marrakech*. His second nonbelletristic book is about the city Tangier. His books are translated into several languages.

In 2018, he published the book about breaking bad news in German, here you find the English version.

The Moment of Encounter—
"Please Come In": *Two People Meet*

Susanne Sieckler waits for her appointment, trying to quell her impatience by glancing through a stack of old magazines. *These must have seen a number of patients already,* she thinks to herself as she flips through the faded pages.

Just 31 years old, Susanne has the feeling, finally, that she has gotten her life back on track. The past years were difficult—immensely difficult—and filled with setbacks: her husband's fatal car accident, the long bouts of grief and despair that followed, not to mention having to care for her two children—Noa, who was only 4 years old at the time, and Melissa, aged 7 years. Then there had been the countless retraining programs that the employment office insisted she attend, none of which had brought steady work. But now, after 4 long years, her kids were finally bringing good grades back from school, she had found a job at a well-respected culinary school on Viktoria-Luise-Platz in the Berlin neighborhood of Schöneberg, and she recently met John, who holds an important position in the solar energy industry.

Then came the diagnosis: "Advanced ovarian cancer, stage IVB—the worst stage possible," the doctor had explained, without her asking. The past half-year had been hell—her exhaustion and stomach pains had long been diagnosed as fatigue syndrome and deemed psychosomatic. And it was not surprising that Susanne Sieckler's body would react to all of the psychological turmoil. An odyssey through various doctors' offices and countless examinations followed, a journey that led only to more uncertainties, not diagnoses. "Why all the abdominal fluid?" the doctors asked again and again. "Do you drink much alcohol?" When a young emergency room doctor first diagnosed her with ovarian cancer, Susanne instantly knew that he was right—she also knew that her life would never be the same.

Today, after 3 months of chemotherapy, it's finally time for the long-planned, long-awaited interim evaluation. "Staging" is the term medical professionals use when making a provisional assessment and evaluation as to whether a tumor has grown smaller or larger. Over the past several months, Susanne has taken two cancer medications, along with a whole host of other prescriptions to make the side effects somewhat bearable. It's halftime—a total of 6 months of chemotherapy are planned—but she can't bring herself to celebrate this milestone. *It's all the same, the important thing is that it worked,* she reasons wearily with herself. The cancer treatment has left its mark, spiritually as well as physically. The shoulder-length, chestnut brown locks that everyone envied Susanne for as a child have vanished. Her eyebrows have fallen out. And she has never gotten used to her physical weakness; even thinking and dreaming are difficult.

Now Susanne is waiting for her doctor, who has promised to discuss the results of the interim evaluation with her today. She hopes with all her heart that the blood counts and computer imaging show positive results, to hear the doctor tell her that the punishing treatment has worked. Before her diagnosis, she had only been to the doctor once, as a 15 year old for tonsillitis. How many times, she wonders, has she had blood drawn since?

She flips through her medical files and counts the laboratory printouts, which resemble secret documents from a numbered bank account: three before the main operation, seven during her stay at the hospital, one before the first dose of chemotherapy, another thirteen over the course of her treatment. She tries to add them together; math has never been her strong suit, but since the chemotherapy it has become even more difficult. After three tries, she has it: *Yesterday was my 23rd blood sampling.* She doesn't know whether to feel proud or sad.

She looks down the white corridor to her left: people come and go, some she knows, others she seems to recognize from somewhere else. She looks at her appointment slip—2:30 P.M.—then up at the clock in the hall—3 P.M. Today she has to go to her daughter's nursery school, where they are organizing a lantern festival, but she has to stop by her house beforehand. In a quiet, friendly voice she asks the nurse if it will be much longer. "I'm sorry Ms. Sieckler," the nurse replies, "your scheduled doctor had a bicycle accident on her way to work and won't be in today. She called right away though, and asked her colleague to speak with you—great, right? Dr. Fernandez-Meier will be with you soon—she's still in an operation, but I imagine she'll be here in just a couple minutes." Susanne doesn't know Dr. Fernandez-Meier, who works in another wing. *It doesn't matter,* Susanne says to herself. *Getting the results today is what matters. Any doctor can give you good news.*

Dr. Fernandez-Meier has practiced medicine for 15 years and is currently pursuing additional training in cancer medicine—she transferred to the cancer center a year ago. On this particular Friday, she is assisting with an extended cancer operation as part of a 24-hour shift, which likely explains why she received a call directly from the polyclinic a little while ago instructing her to take over a colleague's consultation. She is not familiar with the patient's medical history and is not looking forward to the appointment—especially today. She'll manage one way or another. The operation, which lasted over 7 hours, is finally over—they had to remove hundreds of lumps from the abdominal skin, the peritoneum. A 20-cm section of intestine also had to be removed; it had bonded to the ovarian cancer, and the outer layer of tissue was infected with cancerous growth.

It's still early in the day as she makes her way to the polyclinic. She has only 20 minutes to spare for her appointment with Ms. Sieckler, unfortunately, and then has to return to the operating room: a young woman has had a miscarriage and now requires curettage. *Look through the patient's records, get something to drink, have a cereal bar, and call her in,* Dr. Fernandez-Meier thinks to herself, waiting for the elevator. She finds Ms. Sieckler waiting at the door of the consultation room and greets her with a strained smile. "Good morning Ms. Sieckler, I'll be right with you," she says. "Please take your time, catch your breath," Ms. Sieckler replies, trying not to think about her daughter's school festival.

Dr. Fernandez-Meier wrestles with the bottle cap before taking a long sip of water. *Damn, I left the cereal bar in my office,* she thinks, opening the thick file for Ms. Susanne Sieckler, born June 19, 1987. She searches for the clinical report from the first hospital stay and the details of the diagnosis: high-grade papillary serous ovarian carcinoma, FIGO stage IVb; and surgical procedures: lengthwise laparotomy, adenoidectomy, omentectomy, peritonectomy, postoperative remaining tumor smaller than 1 cm.

The doctor recognizes right away that the chances for recovery are not good—tumors remained despite the operation. And then there's the liver metastases. *Hopefully the chemotherapy worked*, she thinks, flipping to the results of the interim evaluation. Tumor marker CA 125 before the chemotherapy, 1490 units; tumor marker CA 125 after three doses of chemotherapy, 2750 units. Dr. Fernandez-Meier frantically searches the PC for the computer tomogram, trying to fend off the suspicion that the tumor has continued to grow after the chemotherapy, to find an argument that will show the difficult cancer treatment wasn't for nothing.

In spite of herself, Dr. Fernandez-Meier grows increasingly impatient. She clicks her tongue and drums her fingers on the tabletop, hoping somehow to speed up time. It's no use; the report is two and a half pages long. She has neither the time nor the patience to read through the entire document—she skips straight to the paragraph titled "General Assessment." Compared to the previous radiological tomograms, "Significant development of peritoneal and hepatic metastases." Her throat goes dry—she can barely swallow. *The tumor has grown, I have to tell her!* she thinks. The telephone rings, the head doctor is on the line and asks her to please show up to the operation room on time, the patient has been waiting for the procedure for a while now. "Yes, of course," she says, and hangs up quickly.

Dr. Fernandez-Meier stands up and looks in the mirror on the door. She quickly wipes off her apricot-colored lipstick—for some reason she feels guilty about wearing the color to deliver such news. She takes a deep breath and opens the door to the waiting room.

"Ms. Sieckler, would you please come in?"

1

Who Needs This Book, and Why a Doctor Had to Write It

CONTENTS

Conveying bad news is one of the most difficult tasks we face, not only as doctors in our everyday clinical work but in practically any profession or sphere of life. But what is bad news, actually? Isn't it much too broad a topic to suggest there is one course of action? Of course, sharing bad news is as varied as life—and death—itself. Still, a couple of general observations can be made. Everybody has some sort of story: doctors, nurses, patients of course, police, medical orderlies, firemen, employers, and even veterinarians. What do these stories hold in common? What can we learn from them, both as recipients and as bearers of bad news?

For those in the medical profession, announcing good news is not a complex challenge in itself, even if we should approach it much more conscientiously than daily practice generally permits. We often communicate good news with even less forethought than is the case with bad news, which is why I address the topic in the second, longer section of the book. Yet, giving a patient bad news without having them collapse into a deep depression—that is truly an art form for doctors. Even in a situation in which things appear "hopeless," one can point out positive aspects about future treatment or the patient's life without glossing over the truth. Successful conversations leave patients feeling adequately informed, supported, and cared for, bringing about a highly satisfying, positive experience for both doctor and patient. For patients facing life-threatening illnesses, an open and empathetic dialogue with their doctor can be an important tool that helps them confront their disease, an existential experience that can later be applied to other areas of their lives.

Breaking Bad News

Sharing bad news has been a common aspect of human interaction for as long as people have been communicating. Cave paintings, for example, were used to indicate that a certain place was not safe, or that a disaster had occurred at that location. Greek mythology tells the story of Apollo, the god of light: When a white crow brought Apollo the news that his lover Coronis had slept with another suitor, Ischys, the god was so enraged that he turned the bird's feathers black forever. He also made it so the crow could no longer sing but only caw. In this case, the bearer of bad news was punished and cursed.

The Old Testament—one of the foundations of the three Abrahamic religions of Judaism, Christianity, and Islam—gives an equally grim account of communicating bad news. In the Book of Job, God subjects his loyal servant, Job, to increasingly unbearable losses and trials, putting Job's relationship with God to a severe test. Today, the proverbial "Job's news" is a metaphor for catastrophic news either that we find to be unjust or which has come out of the blue. At the same time, Job's conversations with his friends, his steadfast faith—what today we might call his spirituality—his resilience, and his steadfast mind also illustrate the various resources humans have at their disposal to help them overcome difficult, even devastating news.

Given the amount of evidence for the important role breaking bad news has played in accompanying and shaping human experience throughout history, it is a minor miracle that we understand so little about how to handle it and that it is discussed so infrequently. The subject is likely too difficult emotionally and too taboo to leave more intimate spheres. To my mind, however, speaking and writing about it seem to be the best ways to do the necessary work of removing the taboo. That is why in addition to chapters with analytical or abstract advice, this book contains sections on what I believe it is that makes up our lives, as well as what it was that brought me to write it in the first place—stories that I either lived through myself or that were told to me. Such stories can give a better impression of what it is that people find difficult about communicating bad news—but also the positive aspects—more than any statistics, tables, or academic studies are able to give. These stories are set apart graphically so they can be found easily. This book can thus also be read as a collection of acute human situations and fates.

I am a person, a father, a husband, a doctor, a scientist, and a teacher; in what follows, I look to share my experiences regarding the subject of bad news and to start a dialogue with you, the reader, as both a doctor as well as a fellow human. I draw especially on 25 years in the medical profession—from my experiences as a young student up to my current position as the director of the Women's Clinic at Berlin's Charité hospital, where I focus on cancerous diseases in women. In sharing my encounters with women patients, their relatives, and my colleagues, I hope to bring the benefit of others' experiences to the table as well. Whether it is as a coworker, the person who is directly affected, or an observer—we see how each of these roles overlap when it comes to communicating bad news. Things rarely have only one meaning, even when a diagnosis seems to. As varied as our occupations may be, different tasks and situations may hold much in common. When I address you as a doctor, patient, relative, or friend, try to put yourself across the table from me and observe your own feelings and thoughts.

But can one actually *learn* how to communicate bad news in the first place, as with diagnosing an illness or performing an operation? A variety of studies have shown that this is in fact the case, and that medical students and doctors alike stand to profit over the long term from engaging with the topic. Bad news may vary greatly—in its frequency, the level of existential threat it implies, as well as any consequences that may result. Sharing bad news is one of the most common but uncomfortable tasks a doctor faces. Over the course of their working life, a doctor will hold maybe over 100,000 conversations with patients and their relatives. Doctors can rely on checklists and professional development curricula that have been certified by recognized medical bodies for nearly every aspect of their everyday work; by contrast, there are few opportunities for continued or advanced training focusing on how one should, or might conduct these conversations. Doctors are required to pursue countless additional qualifications or risk losing their accreditation. Yet, training seminars in doctor–patient communications are not required in Germany, or in any other country for that matter. Conveying bad news is a difficult task for anyone; it is even more difficult when one either seeks to avoid doing so, or conversations remain unreflective because those conducting them have not received professional training.

It is simply not the case that one either does or does not have "the knack" for speaking with people in such a way that when they divulge bad news, the recipient is not stunned by the conversation leaving them feeling totally disoriented and hopeless. It would be better to speak about dialogue, because that is the most important part—a mutual exchange of information. A one-way conversation is doomed to fail and will not permit one's counterpart to begin—or continue—to act independently. What truly matters here is empowering the other person to take responsibility for their own life, to become active so that they don't end up in an emotional and intellectual cul-de-sac.

With "breaking bad news"—a term for which German has still not found an adequate equivalent—I mean communicating a piece of news that will drastically and negatively impact a person's view of the future. From the doctor's perspective, breaking bad news involves a difficult conversation in which the doctor knowingly has to tell a patient that he or she is suffering from a life-threatening, incurable disease. Surely, this definition is not all-encompassing or even generally applicable, as the effect of the news on its recipient can vary widely and may change according to individual factors such as the person's previous experience, life philosophy, spirituality, degree of religious faith, age, and education. A person's cultural context also plays an important role. Then there is the factor of the sum total and frequency of bad news, which can also influence a recipient's attitude toward and perception of the news.

If there has been a succession of bad news, the way a person processes any given conversation depends importantly on how much time has elapsed since the last conversation, the impact the most recent news has had on their life, and/or how successfully previous talks were processed. Especially important for this process, moreover, seems to be recipients' response to bad news. What I mean by this is how actively the person has worked to take charge of their own destiny, and whether the person also received good news during this period. The current state of a person's health is yet another factor whose importance cannot be underestimated. All bad news shares a potential to destroy a person's hopes and dreams; even when this may not match the actual circumstances, it can be taken as such. People may feel threatened, or suddenly confronted with a fundamentally different perspective on their future actions and interests. In my experience, doctors convey bad news much more frequently than they are aware of. Bad news, after all, is not only when a doctor has to tell another person that he or she is incurably ill; it can also be something which from a medical point of view does not represent bad news but still dashes a patient's hopes or triggers fear.

Breaking bad news is a part of many areas of our lives—in the work world as well as the private sphere. Techniques can be learned and professionalized without losing the force of empathy or human interest, and directly learning about how to break bad news while reflecting on the process and training can all help to make this task easier, even fulfilling. This book looks to help readers develop an understanding of this crucial work and to provide both bearers and recipients of bad news with practical aides. My goal is not to devise a patented recipe, according to which each conversation of this sort should proceed, but rather to sort out the essential ingredients of a good conversation, and to develop a sensitivity for how each person—and oneself—might react.

Unbearable Fear

It must have been during my first year of clinical training; I still remember how that spring felt. I was enthralled by gynecology; in particular, complex cancer operations fascinated me. I was continually impressed by people's ability to withstand such invasive operations and diseases.

As a young doctor, I had been assigned the medical station for receiving new admissions, performing anamnesis (when the doctor asks the patient for any medically relevant information), and conducting general examination tests for lung and heart function, after which the head doctor would perform gynecological exams. On that particular day, I was responsible for two new admissions. I asked the nurses if one of the two patients was ready.

"Gerda Müller," said the head nurse, "but hurry up, she's already expected for an EKG." At 86 years old, Gerda Müller was a sight to behold; one never would have guessed her age. I introduced myself and began by asking where she had worked—I was curious to hear about what sort of job would allow one to reach such an age with such beauty. She worked as a secretary for a fashion company. Did she have children? "No, my husband and I didn't want any, there were simply too many other things to do," she replied. "You've always been a non-smoker, right?" I asked. She smiled and nodded. "No, I never smoked." She had been taken into the hospital for vaginal bleeding. "I haven't had my period in over 35 years, so I had curettage and now this diagnosis," she explained, almost as though seeking to excuse herself.

Postmenopausal bleeding is a chief symptom for uterine cancer; curettage also indicated endometrial cancer. Her operation was scheduled for the following day. Every finding pointed toward the early stages of cancer; the good prognosis meant that no additional surgical procedure, such as removal of the lymph nodes, was required.

I asked about her husband. "He's not doing so well. He's 92 and has suffered from asthma for years. Right now his asthma and the pollen are both bothering him, so he stayed at home," she told me. "Our neighbor will stop by later to bring him something to eat—otherwise, Doctor, I do all the housework," she said proudly. "He's no spring chicken," she continued, "so I can't stay in the hospital too long, I have to get back to the house afterward. I hope you'll understand that my husband is really worried about me."

The next day, Gerda was the first patient in the operating room. The operation was a success; her uterus and ovaries were removed without any complications. She remained stable throughout the operation, losing barely any blood, which meant that she could be transferred back directly to her hospital wing.

Then we received a call. It was the neighbor, speaking under her breath. I asked her to speak more loudly, I couldn't understand her. "Mr. Müller is dead," she said. "Dead?" I asked, in disbelief. "Yes dead, he's dead—he shot himself." I called the head doctor immediately and told him the awful story.

"What should I do?" I asked, hoping that he would take everything into his hands, and that I could quickly rid myself of the strange taste in my mouth.

"Call the psychologist please and ask whether he can tell the patient. If you don't get anywhere, you can try me again," he replied.

I called the psychiatrist on duty, who was very kind. I quickly ran through all the details until he interrupted. "Let's slow down, colleague. Where is the patient now?"

"She's doing very well, but she's still in the intensive station because of her age," I answered.

"Does she have relatives?" asked the psychiatrist.

"Yes, a younger sister, but she lives in Düsseldorf and they don't speak often."

"When will she be transferred out of intensive care?"

"Tomorrow, I think," I replied. "What should I do?"

For a second time, I hoped that my colleague would offer to pass on the bad news himself. I waited for him to say something—there was silence on the other end. That unnerved me; I thought maybe the telephone line had cut short. "Hello, are you still there?"

Another pause, and then a sigh.

"I'm here. Please wait until someone who knows the patient can come to the hospital, then ask him or her to take it on," he said, speaking quickly. "You don't have to do that yourself." At the time his words calmed me down, but the strange taste persisted. Was it really not my job? Wasn't this something I *should* be concerned about, after all?

Today, I know that without the responsibility of telling my patients bad news, I could neither love nor fully pursue my job. Over the years, this role has been a gift, allowing me to gather a wonderful set of encounters and experiences both as a doctor and a person. It is something I hope continues into the future.

How Is Communication Taught and Learned?

There is hardly any profession in which communication doesn't play a key role. In medicine, communication is crucial and the backbone of every medical intervention. Yet, in the course of most educational and professional training, verbal communication, much less nonverbal communication, is rarely taught in a structured way. If training does include practice conversations, these only take the form of ideal scenarios rather than real-life situations, and conflict is treated only superficially. In the study of medicine, anamnesis represents a crucial step in diagnosis and prognosis. Despite its unquestionable importance, it receives scant attention in medical education and continued training. The chronic lack of time and face-to-face interaction arising from the everyday pressures of the medical profession places additional pressures on both the quality and quantity of anamnesis.

As before, today, young doctors simply observe the conversational techniques of older doctors without referring to any particular method or reflective process. Just as learning how to play the cello or to ski cannot simply be learned by observation and imitation but must be practiced, new learning and conversational techniques must also be applied and put into practice in medical education and training. While older, experienced doctors have to deal with difficult conversations more frequently, they often pay just as little attention to the needs of patients as their younger colleagues, rarely encouraging them to express their own thoughts and feelings.

Just like certain complicated operation techniques, communicating well—even in situations of grave illness—is a skill that can be learned. Moreover, the positive effects of such training are measurable: patients of doctors who have undergone training in communication show significantly lower levels of stress compared to the patients of a control group of doctors without equivalent training. Unfortunately, to this day, such training rarely forms a requisite component of medical education and training; it is first taught only in regular medical degree courses. All medical professionals—doctors, but also those in care or social services, midwives, psycho-oncologists, and so on—should pursue training in this area, preferably not just once, but at regular intervals.

This consideration applies to any type of person or profession that must reckon with conveying bad news. Police are one obvious example for whom training should focus on situations as difficult as those encountered in medical professions. Once on the train to Leipzig, I struck up a conversation with "Mr. Schmidt," a 50-year-old police officer in uniform. I was interested in his experiences with passing on bad news. Yes, it had been "brought up once during training, and was very important," he replied.

"And do you have to share bad news often?" I continued.

"It depends on your area of responsibility on the force. Earlier, when I was out on patrol it happened two, maybe three times a year. Now I work on the homicide squad, and it happens much more frequently."

I told him about my everyday work as a doctor, he talked about his work as a police officer; we found we shared more in common than not. "It is really damned difficult," I agreed with him wholeheartedly.

"We have an emotional distance though—we don't know the relatives beforehand. As a doctor you've often known the families for a long time. That's a different kind of connection," he reflected.

We discussed the respective advantages and disadvantages of this difference, although in the course of their work, doctors come across any number of situations in which they have to break the news of a death or emergency operation to relatives whom they are meeting for the first time. This is especially common in intensive care. It is difficult to build a relationship with a person you have never met before; often, important background information is lacking not only for the deceased but also for the person with whom one is speaking.

"Still, in medicine and psychology, the relationship between the person sharing the news and the recipient is the backbone for the success of any medical intervention," I said. But it can sometimes help if the person communicating bad news hasn't met their interlocutor and isn't too close to the crisis or drama. "It's good to be aware of these things, but no matter whether we're doctors or police, we can't choose the situations for ourselves. We have to adapt to whatever conditions we find," I said, reflecting on his observations and experiences.

"What happens after the years of training to be police, how have you engaged with the topic over the last 25 years?" I asked.

I was surprised to encounter a long pause, considering that up to that point in our conversation he had answered my questions clearly and in great detail. "Subsequent training happens on an as-needed basis," he replied, hesitantly.

"On an as-needed basis? I don't understand," I countered, and asked him to explain.

"It means that a police officer can be retrained if he expresses a need for it, but otherwise he has to decide for himself."

"There's yet another similarity—and difference—with the medical profession," I said. "After medical training, the topic isn't approached in a structured manner either, that's the similarity."

"And the difference?"

"At the hospital or doctor's office, the doctor has to organize opportunities for further training himself and generally pay out of pocket, even if the health insurance companies and especially the patients stand to benefit."

It is my opinion that professions such as the police or medicine should take a very different approach to the subject of "breaking bad news" than they currently do. Everyone talks about safety and prevention and then forgets when it comes to such a critical topic. In medicine, countless areas such as hygiene, radiation protection, work safety, and blood transfusions are subject to regular, obligatory training sessions. Courses are also required for any number of certifications. Why, then, is there no education or training on how to handle bad news? At the very least, a methodical query among relevant types of profession might help. On principal, continued education courses should also be free for participants.

Meanwhile, I have initiated a seminar with commissioners and doctors. The feedback of the attendees was great; there were more similarities than differences, despite the different working fields. Both professions underlined that they have learned from the other groups and that the view on the other profession helps to reflect his own field.

Agadir

It's 9 P.M. I call my assistant: I want to visit my patients at Station 35 one final time before leaving—I hope—the next morning for 7 long days in Agadir, Morocco, with my family. There is a teacher from Libya at the station; a frightened patient with a suspected case of ovarian cancer who lies in another room. The second patient is currently suffering from a number of difficult secondary illnesses that make an operation too risky; we are trying to resolve a number of internal medical problems. We proceed to the neighboring room, where an older patient is recovering from her operation of a few days before. We find her in surprisingly good shape and in an excellent mood. The neighboring patient was also operated on several days ago, for over 5 hours. Both are happy to see us.

"Doctor, what did they actually operate on?" I hear the younger patient ask as I speak with the older patient. I look over, somewhat irritated; the operation was 6 days ago already and I have discussed it with her. Before I can answer, my young assistant jumps in: "The uterus, the ovaries, abdominal skin folds, the omental sac, and lymph nodes—just as we had agreed on before the operation, and as I've explained several times, including this morning."

"I know, but it can't be all that bad, everything will be fine—right, Doctor?" the patient pleads, looking up at me with her hand outstretched. I take her hand in mine, explaining that we have to wait until after the tissue analysis before we can discuss.

"The results aren't in yet?" she asks. I look to my assistant, who replies that they will probably come in the next few days. We say goodbye to both patients. A few steps outside the room, my assistant turns to me: "Doctor, she is so likable, but she simply won't accept a cancer diagnosis. She keeps hoping against hope that it's a benign tumor, but the histology is there—it's ovarian cancer, we're just missing a few additional tests. I'd rather wait until we have all the findings and then I'll tell her."

I stop. "It's not good to put off telling the truth and then spend valuable energy concealing it. Patients notice this sort of thing. Let's go back in," I say.

"Now, doctor?" she asks, shocked.

"Yes," I answer, "now."

We open the door and both patients light up, as though we were coming back to celebrate a birthday. I sit down beside the patient, take her hand in mine, and briefly explain again what we operated on. Then I tell her that the results have come back and that she has ovarian cancer. We have to wait, however, for further test results from the lymph nodes and the peritoneum to determine exactly what state the tumor is in.

"Of course, doctor—we'll wait for the final results, that's alright," she replies. I tell her that it's important to me that she knows the results so that she can get her bearings. On the way out the door, she calls to me: "But Doctor, I won't need chemotherapy, right?"

"I don't know that yet, but most women do need chemotherapy, so please assume that in several weeks we'll begin a cancer treatment with drug therapy. But we can't say yet." And that was how I ended my shift on that particular evening.

We've been on the Atlantic coast for several days now, finally escaping from under the gray skies of Berlin to enjoy the luxurious November sun over the port town of Agadir in southern Morocco. We watch the gulls fly along the horizon—for some reason they keep moving in a circle, more than a hundred of them wheeling about on a funny sort of carousel, unconcerned about whether they have the best seat on the ride. We meet Nizar, smiling, the chef d'animation, his dark hair gelled back in a wild tangle. Nizar is a true jack-of-all-trades: he can sing, dance salsa, surf, play piano and guitar, and speak German, Arabic, English, Spanish, French, and Moroccan—all that at only 36 years old. Back in Morocco for 9 months now, his wife Tamara is pregnant; two other children remain with his ex-wife in Switzerland. Every time we come across Nizar, he's either smiling or singing. On meeting, we quickly became friends, and over the years a trusting relationship has developed. He left Morocco as a young man to pursue his artistic talents in hotels the world over, to delight audiences no matter how large or small. He performed on stages in Algeria, Tunisia, Cuba, and Egypt before arriving in Switzerland and finding work as a train engineer.

Egypt proved to be a dramatic turning point in his young life. Racing through the streets of Sharm el-Sheikh one day on his motorbike, two women suddenly stepped out in front of a tour bus to cross the street. Nizar couldn't have seen them coming; he spent the following 4 weeks in a coma with severe brain damage and knee injury. Fortunately, he had been wearing a helmet despite the blazing heat, which probably saved his life. When he finally woke, he thought that he was lying in his own bed and had overslept and would now be late for his job at the hotel "Ali Baba." Then he realized that the room was painted entirely white, and that his sister was sitting by his side. "But she lives in Casablanca," Nazar thought to himself, "that's almost 5000 km away. How can that be?" His sister Amal told him what had happened, crying from happiness and grief at the same time, he could tell. "Nizar, there's something else

I have to tell you," her crying intensified, and her voice dropped. "The two women crossing in front of the bus—they're dead, brother, I'm sorry, but they died." Nizar didn't answer; he had heard the bad news but could neither understand nor believe it.

For that entire day and night, Nizar didn't speak; he kept hoping somehow to wake up out of what was surely a horrible dream. At some point, the medical staff also learned that Nizar had woken up from his coma. Just a few minutes later, after a brief examination by a silent, heavyset doctor who shone a weak flashlight into his eyes and looked down his throat with a small brass spoon, Nizar was taken into custody by soldiers and transferred to a building at the edge of the city district. The two women were from Germany, the incident was politically sensitive and had yet to be explained sufficiently, the soldiers told him. For the time being, Nizar had to go to jail while the court decided.

Nizar's jail cell had three tiny windows. Although he spoke excellent Arabic, Nizar insisted on speaking English; he didn't want to speak in Arabic. Walking was the only thing that kept him alive during that period, he told me. "I walked constantly: around my narrow cell, the dusty courtyard, the dirty showers. I would have gone crazy otherwise." He was held a total of 5 months until he was finally released and allowed to travel to friends in Switzerland. With medical help and his friends' support, he sought to heal from his physical and spiritual wounds. He also sought to make a new start, marrying a Swiss woman and leaving behind the hotel life that seemed so inauthentic at points, more like a circus show. He studied to be a train engineer. But now he is back in Agadir, and he has come to love his work again. He dances, sings, plays, does acrobatics—interacting with so many people makes him feel alive, and hotels are where he truly feels at home. "And what helped you to overcome this tragedy?" I asked him. "Time and space to love my own heart again," Nizar answered.

A Topic That Affects Us All—Even in Private

Just several weeks ago at an academic conference in Berlin, I met a colleague from Casablanca, in Morocco; he researches vaccinations for infectious children's diseases. We immediately took to one another, and he soon confided with me that he had lost his younger brother and his brother's wife in the terror attacks in Nice, France, on July 14, 2016. I asked who had brought him the news. "Their sons were able to save themselves at the last minute from the truck. They called my daughter that evening. They had been close friends ever since they were young, almost like siblings. It helped a lot that we didn't find out from people we didn't know," he replied, his voice trembling.

This book talks a lot about medicine, doctors, the hospital, and treatment. I'm a doctor after all, and most of my experiences with the art of conveying difficult news come from my professional environment. Yet, I am also a father, husband, brother, son, colleague, and friend. I know a lot of people; I like people and their stories. Maybe that's why I've also come across a number of stories from outside the hospital that also belong in this book. This book is about life in all its diversity, not just the life of a doctor. What's more, I want to be personable—over the course of the following chapters, I will often ask you as a reader to open yourself emotionally and to risk vulnerability when you have bad news to share with someone. For communication to be even-handed, it must always, always, always be an exchange—otherwise it remains a one-way street. For that reason, too, I share highly personal thoughts and stories of my own.

Stories like the following: We meet with our friends Andreas and Özlem; they've invited us to dinner in Potsdam. Andreas has worked as a pilot for a number of years; Özlem is a stewardess. Our children are just about the same age and love playing together. The dinner is elaborate, the mood boisterous, and we're delighted to be in each other's company again—the last time must have been 3 months ago already. Each time we meet, I pester Andreas with questions about flying safety in the belief that somehow it will allay my constant fear of flying. And somehow we get on the subject of his father, a sports teacher who lived a healthy life, loved tennis and golf, and went jogging multiple times a week.

In 2010, Andreas was scheduled for a flight to the Dominican Republic and took the rare opportunity to invite his parents and wife at the time to spend a couple of relaxing days taking in the azure blue sky, white sand, and bottle-green sea. Like his father, Andreas also enjoys sports—he loves to run for kilometers and to climb.

The first day of their vacation, Andreas recalled, he had more difficulty than usual with his running, maybe from the turbulent flight of the previous day. After about 2 hours, he came back to the bungalow, where his mother was waiting for him. "What's wrong mother?" he asked. She didn't reply. "Mom, what is it?" Andreas repeated. "Andreas, your father died—he was lying there in bed, I thought he was just sleeping deeply, he had been there for so long."

Andreas broke off. "It was probably a heart attack—all of his brothers had heart attacks," he continued. "I couldn't understand it. He had been to the doctor just days before, who gave him top marks for his health. And now he was dead, how could that even be?"

"What happened then?" I asked. "I had to handle all the formalities," he replied, "all without being able to speak a word of Spanish. Cash in hand settled whatever laws had to be observed, though; otherwise it might have taken weeks to bring my father back to Germany. I also had to postpone my return flight—I called the captain for our crew and told him what had happened. 'Great, now where am I supposed to find another copilot?' was his answer. 'I'll find one,' I replied, then hung up before I got too worked up. I switched shifts with a colleague from another team, and actually managed to get all the necessary documents together so I could be there with my mother and father on the trip back."

"You swapped places with the colleague but you weren't flying as a copilot, right?" I asked, expecting a simple no. "Wrong!" answered Andreas. "That helped—as a copilot I could just slip into the work and forget about it. I wouldn't have been able to sit there by my mother as she wept on the plane."

"And you were actually able to focus on the flight, on your work?' I asked again.

"I couldn't block every thought, but believe me, I did my job just like I had on hundreds of flights before. It was only when I got home and took off my uniform that I really began to feel and to realize that I had lost my dad. I called up my sister and told her about the accident. I cried the whole night and then, the next awful morning, I somehow found the strength to organize the burial."

"Sometimes routine can help" I told him, then thanked him for his openness. "Yes, but today I regret the fact that I didn't stay by my mother's side the whole time." "And did you ever tell her that?" I asked. "No, maybe I should, maybe..." "What helped your mother?" I let myself ask. "Her family and her faith. She always talks about that poem by Thornton Wilder—I don't know it word for word but I'll try: 'There is a land of the living and a land of the dead and the bridge is love, the only survival, the only meaning.'"

2

Breaking Bad News Well

CONTENTS

As I suggested earlier, techniques for breaking bad news well can be learned, just as an athlete trains for a 400-meter race, a policeman quickly learns to recognize false bank notes or a doctor learns to perform an emergency hemorrhage operation. As with any learning process, one's attitude, willingness, and desire to learn are all preconditions to success. Please take a moment now and quietly say to yourself: "I want to learn." With short anecdotes from my practical experience, I want to support you in this position—I also encourage you to reflect on your own experiences and observations while reading.

A Visit from the Head Doctor

Whether it was during a stay at the hospital ourselves or having watched any number of TV series, we've all been there before: the head doctor's visit. The visit is rarely a good moment to communicate bad news; the visits are generally more reminiscent of a small presentation, even if at first it is unclear what exactly all the fuss is about. The vaguely threatening wash of white coats; the numerous assistants, senior physicians, and nurses thronging around the head doctor; the palpable rush of time—none are ideal conditions for discussing complex topics in depth. This is especially the case as the assistants are largely focused, as they often are, on presenting all the details of a patient's history to the head doctor without making any errors or leaving anything out. Personally, I ask for the patient's results *before* opening the door to the patient's room.

Another fact that makes an eye-to-eye conversation more difficult in a literal sense is that many patients are either lying or sitting down. In spite of their frequent rush for time, some doctors try to put this to rights by sitting down at their patient's bed before beginning to speak. To protect the confidence of the conversation—also from neighboring patients—others invite patients into a separate room. I've found it valuable to visit the patient in their own room, as the patient's immediate environment provides a great deal of information. There's the patient's favorite book on the nightstand, for example, next to her newspaper of choice and pictures of her relatives. It's also interesting to observe what relations and friends have brought along: flowers, drinks, a grandson's paintings, or good luck charms. Each detail provides important insight into the patient's situation. During my weekly visits, I look, on the one hand, to identify real medical problems and to determine suitable diagnostic and therapeutic measures with my colleagues. On the other hand, I try to give the patient the feeling that our team truly cares for her, and to respect each patient's individuality as well as the person who lies behind the diagnosis. In doing so, it is more about attitude than it is the right words—in my opinion, a head doctor's visit can just as well be a time for laughter or a moment to reflect on nonmedical subjects.

An Afternoon Walk

Ms. Holler arrives at my office breathing somewhat heavily, and takes longer than usual to find her seat. We've known each other for some years now; the pauses in between her treatments have grown shorter and shorter as the cancer has progressed. She finally takes a seat on the black chair, still feeling her final climb up the stairs. The tumor markers from the computed tomography (CT) scan show that the cancer has continued to grow despite the recent chemotherapy. Just 2 days ago, she had to go to the emergency room for increased stomach pain; cancerous peritoneal nodes had caused various restrictions in her intestine, preventing it from functioning normally. The restrictions and increased gas buildup caused the intestines to expand so greatly that one could feel them through the hard abdominal wall—fortunately, enemas had helped. She didn't want to stay in the hospital and returned home afterward; she is returning now for a consultation because she wants to speak right away about the next steps.

"We've known each other for 4 years, Doctor, you know that, right?" she says to me, smiling. Smiling has always come easy to her. I feel her stomach, which is significantly softer than it has been in the past several days. Still, we both decide that it's better for her to return to the hospital for several tests: her heavy breathing means that there is water in her pleural cavity that should be drained, while the radiological examination of her gastrointestinal tract should provide a clearer idea of what state the intestinal restrictions are in.

Ms. Holler and I get along well; she always finishes our meetings with a soft "*obrigada*," which means "thanks" in Portuguese. Although she can't actually speak any Portuguese—or Spanish for that matter—I still remember our third meeting, when I found out where she knew *obrigada* from. "It's because my father is Brazilian," she answered, much to my surprise.

"Your father is Brazilian," I repeated in disbelief.

"That's right," she said. "He's fairly famous there, I'm his illegitimate child. We're in touch by writing, but I haven't seen him for over 50 years. Unfortunately, he can't visit me or invite me there due to his position, but we're in touch and that makes me happy."

"How's your father?" I ask her.

"I don't know, I haven't been able to talk to him for weeks. Whenever I call someone who I don't know and can't understand picks up."

"If you'd like, I can ask one of my colleagues if she can call and ask about your father," I suggest. Her beautiful smile returns, and she nods earnestly. My secretary knocks gently at the door to tell me that a young assistant who is set to accompany me while admitting a new patient has arrived as scheduled and wants to outline the patient's relevant medical information. I show the assistant in and ask if she would sit down with us briefly. She looks somewhat unsure but takes a seat.

"Ms. Holler, what is the worst piece of news you have ever received in your life?" I asked.

"My cancer diagnosis," she answers quickly.

"The first diagnosis or the recurrence, when the cancer returned after the operation and chemotherapy?"

"The first diagnosis!" she answers again, without thinking twice.

"How did the doctor act when she told you?" I continue.

"It was really bad. I still remember it like it was yesterday. She told me that my stomach was full of cancerous growths. During the ultrasound, she kept saying: 'There's cancer, here too, and there, and there too,' and just shaking her head, with her large earrings jangling. I sat there staring at the eerie black and white images on the monitor and thinking to myself 'The cancer is taking away all the white space inside of me, it's stealing the light from my life.'"

"What kind of feeling did that leave you with?"

"The doctor and I both felt totally hopeless. There was no plan, no idea how we should, or could proceed. The only thing she told me was that I had to get to a hospital as quickly as possible, nothing else. No address, no recommendation, nothing."

"What did you do?"

"I went to my office, closed out the final pension requests for our policyholders, and said goodbye to my colleagues. I couldn't reach my boss, so I left her a message. I thought I would never be back there."

"So when you left the doctor's office you went straight to work and not to a friend, or simply somewhere you could be alone?" I asked, amazed.

"I called a friend, but it was also clear to me that I had to go back to work. I had only excused myself for 2 hours, and I had to process the requests."

"And then?"

"Then my friend arrived, and we took a really lovely walk along the Spree River. I remember well how gorgeous it was—a picture-perfect spring day. We walked along together, not even saying all that much. Just walking with someone can bring you closer. It was so beautiful; I'd never seen such pretty birds before. There was even a goldfinch with a red face, white head, and ivory beak. It's considered a symbol for Christ's Passion because it loves thistles."

"And what helped you the most to process the difficult diagnosis of advanced cancer?" I wanted to know.

"My friend—I was so grateful to her. She showed up right away and just listened. And she did that even though we had fought over some insignificant matter several weeks before, and today we aren't in touch. Her listening gave me the feeling that I mattered, that our friendship was stronger than either of us suspected. Without her I may not have made the appointment at the hospital. She accompanied me and day by day, the situation became more bearable and hopeful."

As Ms. Holler makes her way out of my office, she pauses for a moment in the doorway, then softly murmurs "*obrigada*." "*Obrigado*," I reply.

Preparing for an Existential Conversation

The conversation between patient and doctor matters as much as it does because it is the only way to counteract fear. As such, it is probably the most important medicine a doctor can offer. As one patient put it, "The only thing that helped was speaking with my doctor or relatives. Without the conversations, the monster of cancer grew in size each day; with them the monster shrank."

But what does the art of conducting a difficult conversation actually consist of? The patient should be told early on that an explanatory meeting will take place as soon as possible after the key test results have returned, with the time for the meeting given as precisely as possible so that the patient has time to notify their relatives or write down questions. This relieves patients from the stress of trying to intercept the doctor in the hallway or get hints from a nurse. To put it concretely: give advance notice of the conversation and the potential content with something like the following: "I'd like to meet with you this afternoon around … o'clock so we can talk about the test results in peace." It may be preferable to make two appointments; decisions shouldn't have to be made all at once. Again, this relieves stress—for all parties. In the hospital, it is not advisable to schedule appointments too late in the day or on Friday afternoons. At the office it is generally better to schedule appointments outside of visiting hours, as one is more at ease. Spend time preparing: Are all the results in? Am I familiar with the patient's history? Do I have the right patient? Is the diagnosis correct? To err is human and mistakes happen—they can also place the patient's psyche under terrible stress. Are the main topics of the conversation clear in my mind? Do I know how I want to begin the conversation? Pause for a moment, hold, and breathe deeply.

Experiences from dedicated workshops and everyday clinical practice show that good communication is not only learnable but can also improve a doctor's feeling of satisfaction with their own work. For their part, patients feel respected, and their compliance improves accordingly. By compliance, I mean a patient's level of cooperation with a recommended set of medical measures. In general, good compliance means that recommendations are followed. Difficult conversations pose one of the greatest challenges to the doctor's relationships with patients and relatives alike. At the same time, breaking bad news is one of the most common activities a doctor faces. Within the scope of my own daily work, "bad news" often addresses women dealing with severe cases of cancer and their relatives, although an unrealized wish for children or miscarriages can also present extremely difficult situations for everyone involved. Conversations addressing something that is either incurable or no longer possible tend to take on another dimension that can be very challenging.

Most patients look for open and honest communication that leaves them with a reasonable degree of hope. Placing ourselves in the patient's situation, doctors—most of us at least—would similarly prefer to be told honestly if we had an illness.

A "difficult conversation" between patient and doctor that is satisfying to both parties depends on any number of factors, many of which are easily influenced. Much can be accomplished through sufficient preparation. Aside from that, it is also about recognizing the patient's needs, active listening, asking the right questions, having the courage to pause, making sure the patient understands their general situation and test results, not fearing emotions, and understanding the gradual nature of the conversation.

Then there's the most important part: taking time to visualize the beginning of the conversation, the conversation itself, and what will come after. Doctors should treat intake conversations as a foundation for establishing trust. The first impression is especially important, as it is the most sensitive part of the conversation. A comprehensive anamnesis will include questions not only about the patient's professional background, but also romantic and family life and general living situation. It is the most important diagnostic measure there is, not only giving doctors information about medical and social factors, but also providing doctors with important insights into the patient's psyche, mood, and feelings. If you learn during the first conversation that the patient has a difficult relationship with her husband, you will better understand why she wouldn't want him to be there for a consultation. Does the patient have a partner who is sick or in need of care, elderly parents, or (young) children? Who and what else will be affected in the event of a negative test result and the prescribed treatment?

In recent years, a wide range of researchers, doctors, and psychologists have taken an interest in how to communicate bad news, and some have released initial publications on the subject. One particularly popular model is the "SPIKES" system developed by Walter Baile. In addition to being a doctor and psychologist at the University of Texas MD Anderson Cancer Center, one of the world's largest facilities of its kind, Baile is a professor of behavioral research and psychiatry as well as the director of the center's I*Care program. He developed the following model based on his own experience and various scientific studies.

Baile distinguishes between the following six steps:

1. S—Setting Up the Interview
2. P—Assessing Patient's Perception
3. I—Obtaining the Patient's Invitation
4. K—Giving Knowledge and Information
5. E—Addressing the Patient's Emotions
6. S—Providing Strategy and Summary

I have incorporated Baile's system into my own work, and it plays an important role in my considerations when preparing for and conducting effective conversations. The steps do not need to be followed mindlessly—I also follow my own lead at times, responding to the situation as it changes. Nevertheless, the SPIKES method can serve as a useful, but above all easily remembered set of guidelines. First, however, let's take a step back to remind ourselves that it's never simply our own thoughts we need to keep in mind but an additional perspective as well—in this case, patients and their relatives.

What Do Patients Expect of a Good Doctor?

Patients hold many expectations of their doctors. Aside from professional competence, three crucial properties are openness, patience, and an ability to give encouragement. "I need ideas about how to overcome my illness, rather than simply wallowing in the disease," as one patient put it when I broke the news of her cancer's advance following a third round of chemotherapy. If you replace the word "patient" in the title of this section with the word "human," the matter becomes somewhat clearer. People expect consideration and assistance, not simply a diagnosis or an operation. When communicating bad news to someone, try to give that person the feeling that they are in a protected space with you, a space where it's possible to express personal thoughts and feelings.

To do so, preparation is key—the "setting up," or first "S" in Walter Baile's SPIKES sequence. As explained previously, this essentially means getting a handle on the conditions surrounding the conversation. While the patient's immediate environment can provide a number of important clues at the outset, you can also make additional inquiries. A doctor can consult with one of the nurses or assistants, for example, who are often in much closer and longer contact with patients than are doctors through "brief" consultations, which usually fall outside the context of doctor–patient meetings, and who may provide helpful insights into patients' lives, thoughts, and emotions. Questions like the following can prove useful: What helps the patient? What has helped her before to overcome difficult life moments or crises? What people were important to her at the time? These questions may help clarify, for example, the potential impact of bad news and its consequences on the patient's partnership or other relationships.

The social dimension of health—contact with other people—is widely recognized as an important foundation for "multidimensional health," which the World Health Organization (WHO) defined in 1947 as: "a state of complete physical, mental, and social well-being." Even though this aspect is generally overlooked when it comes to communicating bad news, it is precisely what matters. It shows that health and sickness both have various dimensions that are of fundamental importance to developing an "overall picture" or assessment, and that one continually needs to observe and operate at different levels when dealing with crises. The social environment plays a particularly important role here, a context that the everyday world rarely grants the attention it deserves.

One current study shows, for example, that cancer patients who live with their partners have significantly better prognoses than single cancer patients. This effect is even stronger among men than it is women. In the study, radiation oncologist Ayal Aizer of the Brigham and Women's Hospital in Boston, Massachusetts, evaluated data from the U.S. Cancer Registry for over 700,000 patients suffering from the most common forms of the disease, such as lung, intestinal, and breast cancers. Aizer observed that the disease often made less progress among cancer patients who were married than among patients who lived alone.

The factor of time, that is, fixing a concrete appointment for the conversation, is another extraordinarily important detail. Patients should generally be told early on that they will be apprised of the good or bad news as soon as possible after all the essential findings have come back. Time and again, I have observed how doctors put off making appointments on the pretext that the test results are not in yet, even though they are. Often, the real reason is that they have not yet determined a treatment strategy in consultation with the senior physician or at a Tumor Conference.* However, one does not necessarily need to have reached a decision regarding treatment in order to communicate difficult news. In this case, communicating the results is what matters, not an immediate treatment plan. This applies for good news as well as bad news. Granted, it will certainly be easier if treatment options can be floated as a sort of lifeline.

I would like to remind readers, however, that a patient's ability to absorb anymore information will in any event be severely limited once bad news has been delivered. Following a bad diagnosis or prognosis, it is more about orientation than it is detailed facts such as dosage or the specific side effects of various treatment plans. As has been shown, patients won't be able to take much in. It will take time, and potentially another conversation before treatment options can be discussed reasonably, and you can begin to make decisions together.

Splitting the conversation into two—one without a treatment plan, followed by one with a treatment plan—can remove uncomfortable pressure on all sides: not only for patients and their relatives, but also for doctors and nurses. Unfortunately, although nurses are usually the direct point of contact for patients, they are rarely present at the doctor–patient conversation and must therefore regularly dodge patients' questions about treatment. Many doctors seem to believe it is better to tell the patient "everything," maybe for fear of forgetting something, even if it is a tiny detail. In doing so, they confuse an announcement, information, and explanation. Initially, all that matters is communicating the message that allows for the next practical step—nothing more, and nothing less.

More than 80% of patients wish for a caregiver of their choosing to be present during these conversations, yet more than 80% of patients learn about their test results and receive news of their cancer diagnosis alone. That being the case, it seems obvious to ask patients ahead of time whether they would like to have someone accompany them for the conversation. It should also obviously be respected if this isn't the case. Furthermore, it's important to remember with bad news that one's basic role is constantly changing: The person receiving the news will soon be the one communicating it when that person shares it with their partner, children, or friends. It could be compared to a relay race, in which the bad news is passed on from one to the next.

Before the first words of bad news are uttered, it is vital to understand how the recipient is currently feeling, and thus prepare them ahead of time—both in terms of content and emotionally—for the situation at hand. That is the "P" in Baile's method: "Assessing Patient's Perception." In other words, where does the patient perceive herself to be, what emotional and psychological awareness does she have of her

---

* A Tumor Conference is a meeting among various technical specialists from the branches of cancer medicine, radiation therapy, and pathology that usually occurs once a week, in which all the medical findings are evaluated and a treatment plan is established.

illness? Specifically, it may be helpful to feel out the current state of your counterpart's knowledge, her emotional state, and expectations. This "search" shouldn't take too much time however, as patients generally have a feeling they are about to receive bad, or at least important news. Patients should not be underestimated.

I've often had the feeling while observing these talks that—more or less consciously, whether it is from insecurity or excessive caution—the doctor is trying to slow the pace of the conversation, not only in their speech but also the rate at which he or she delivers information. For their part, patients are often "hungry" for the truth. Right speech—and this also literally means one's pronunciation—lies at the heart of a good doctor–patient conversation. Pay close attention to your phrases and expressions; a doctor's vocabulary can be intimidating to patients and their relatives, often sounding like spy agency lingo. For this reason, it is best not to use foreign words in such conversations. Having to explain what you've just said often unnecessarily lengthens the conversation, generally at the expense of the patient's focus on its essential aspects. Unfortunately, the way in which medical results are described can also lead to fundamental misunderstandings in interpretation. Take "positive results," for example: to patients, this may sound like recovery, while doctors often take this to mean results that confirm the presence of an illness. A test for a highly infectious disease is "positive" in medicine if the pathogen or the antibody shows up in the patient's blood—anything but a good result. In training sessions, doctors and students should practice describing negative news as "negative" and positive medical results as "positive."

All in all, great sensitivity is required to discern how much a patient actually knows. Obviously, it shouldn't feel at all like an interrogation. In my discussions with colleagues, I hear repeatedly about patients who have been sick for a long time already and had countless conversations about their illness, and who are then heard to say, "Unfortunately, I don't really know anything, I haven't spoken with a doctor about it." Especially if they took part in one of these conversations, doctors may feel hurt or angry. They have already taken a great deal of time on the patient from their perspective—time that they often didn't have anyway, or which was then lost on other patients. It isn't necessary to take a patient's momentary impression to heart, however. Instead, one should simply accept the fact that the patient needs to talk more, that it has not been easy for them to understand all this. And how could it be? The news has barged in on the patient's life and left their life plans in disarray. In such cases, it can be helpful to remember the guiding principle that "it is not about what was said, it is about what the patient heard." The recipient's subjective perception is decisive for anyone communicating bad news to another person. When a patient says that he or she "doesn't know," this may be an appeal for more contact and attention, or may even partially express an unconscious repression, a defense mechanism used to overcome the disease.

The doctor should prepare for a conversation much like a professional skier visualizes the course in his mind before a run down a mountain. When doing so, it's important to pay particular attention to the beginning and the end, and to look for the good in the bad. Doctors often enter these conversations as if from another world—the operating room or a conversation with another patient, as in the story at the beginning of the book with Susanne Sieckler and Dr. Fernandez-Meier. This isn't a rare occurrence but a part of everyday life in hospitals and doctors' offices. In order to prepare for the task at hand and be fully present, it can help to stop and take a moment and/or perform a little ritual. Some colleagues, for example, wash their hands as they do before an operation, in order to "wash off" whatever it was they were doing before and to prepare for the upcoming conversation. One colleague told me she takes 10 deep breaths. Another lights a cigarette and takes several minutes to himself. Another told me that she has a ritual of looking out the window and simply observing the flow of life on the street, both in order to ground herself and to reassure herself that the earth will continue to turn even after the conversation.

It isn't necessary to overthink the seating arrangement for the conversation; it is enough to make sure that loud or disturbing noises or people who are not involved won't interrupt you. Ideally, hospitals should have a dedicated room for these types of conversation; most patients stay in multiple-bed rooms, where it would hardly be appropriate to have such an important discussion. If the conversation takes place at the doctor's office, the consultation room is adequate. A special room isn't necessary— with the right preparation, any room can work. Advisers on how to stage these conversations often like to suggest avoiding an arrangement in which the doctor sits directly across from the patient, as this can lend a confrontational aspect. Instead, one might sit diagonally across the table from the patient, to be able to turn toward the patient more easily and prevent the impression that one is putting up a wall or border. It is not necessary to maintain steady eye contact, although you can if you prefer. Sitting diagonally is also more conducive to creating a feeling of connection. Neither the design nor the height of the chairs should vary too greatly, so that both parties can see eye to eye.

I have spent years listening to such recommendations at seminars or lectures in large auditoriums. At first, I strictly observed each, until gradually I trusted myself to alter them, or even leave some out. In the meantime, I've developed considerable doubts about their value, as in my opinion it is not the seating or the right furniture that matters but rather that the person to whom one is speaking really feels comfortable. A "traditional seating" arrangement, for example, in which the patient sits on one side of the desk and the doctor on the other in a consulting room, can absolutely bring the patient a sense of security. I still recall inviting one patient into a separate room as a young doctor in order to tell her about unfavorable prognostic findings from a histological exam—at the time, the neighboring patient's extended family was visiting. The blinding white room was entirely empty; it was used as a storage space for IV poles. As I opened the door, the patient, whom I had known for some time, said: "Doctor, what is it? The results must be really bad, right?" It was as though she had caught me stealing apples. "How did you get that idea?" I replied. "Because you've never called me out of the room before," she answered. If I had thought through the preparation ahead of time as described previously, I could have spared her feeling of dread and made it easier to breach the subject.

Time and again, doctors ask me if they should touch their patients when sharing bad news. It's a question that can't be answered with a simple "Yes" or "No," as it depends on a variety of factors and the individual situation. In particular, the person communicating the bad news should ask himself if the patient would be comfortable with that in the first place—have I had physical contact with the patient before? How did the patient react, for example, when I took his arm at a recent meeting? It should be respected if the patient prefers not to be touched physically; doctors need not feel aggrieved. One compromise might involve setting out paper tissues on the table to offer to the patient if he needs; many take this as a sympathetic, even physical gesture. As with every part of an existential conversation, one's own knowledge and experience matter. These are no substitute, however, for putting oneself in the recipient's place. While this takes times, it also pays great dividends—for both sides. As a rule, when patients try to place themselves in their doctor's position, their conversations and relationship improve.

Try and develop a feeling for whether the person with whom you are sharing bad news is ready to receive it, and how much preliminary conversation is necessary before getting to the heart of the matter. Be respectful, but never underestimate your counterpart. How would you like to receive this news? Let different scenarios play out in your mind without fixing a specific course. What do they look like? That is the "I" in the SPIKES model (Obtaining the Patient's Invitation), in other words first internally, and then actually inviting the patient into the dialogue and giving the patient a feeling for the aim of the discussion.

The "K" stands for "Giving Knowledge and Information" to the patient. In this case, it is about giving warning signs before actually delivering news of the negative prognosis. It may be a sentence expressing one's regret, a somber look, or both. What is important is that the signal is given clearly, and that it lands with the patient. Only then can the actual medical information follow.

It is possible to stay factual and truthful while remaining empathetic and without diluting the content of the message to be delivered. Try to figure out your counterpart's emotions but also respect them, without rushing to judgment. Try to make the protected sphere of your conversation larger and more secure and make room for the emotions of the person receiving the bad news. Grief or rage, despair, concern for others, self-pity, bitterness, even humor: not only are all these permitted, given the situation, they are absolutely normal. Taking in the person's feelings, and in cases reflecting them back is the "E" in SPIKES: "Addressing the Patient's Emotions" with empathic responses.

There is still the final "S," which stands for "Strategy and Summary." Depending on the situation, at the end of the conversation try and summarize the overall state of affairs. The summary shouldn't be a long monologue, but rather a distillation of what you've discussed. One or two sentences are often enough. The patient should take mental note of them, as should you—they are potential building blocks for subsequent conversations.

As I mentioned, the SPIKES model should not be followed unthinkingly but serve only as a guide. Anyone communicating difficult, even devastating news, needs a foundation from which to operate and get their bearings for the difficult conversation ahead. Such a foundation also makes the person sharing the news less afraid of the conversation. A certain amount of fear can help to keep one sensitive and attentive however, and we must accept it as an essential part of the task. Every conversation is different: one cannot simply use the same format repeatedly and assume that everything will be fine. Still, in the course of my own work as well as that of many colleagues, there are a number of experiences that have been indispensable, at least for me, and whose particular importance I would like to emphasize. These crucial aspects come up regularly at lectures or seminars when I speak with police or other doctors and students about the art of communicating bad news.

Being Aware of One's Role

On the way to my office on the first floor of the hospital, I meet my assistant: Dr. Fernandez-Meier has just come back from vacation. Her mother is very ill. As the only child of seven living and working abroad, she provides a great deal of support to her family in Peru, helping out as much as she is able emotionally, but also financially. Today she's back at work, explaining a planned chemotherapy to a patient.

One wouldn't know just from looking at her that she is worried as she smiles and tries to answer all the patient's questions: "What can I do about my weakness? Will I even be able to withstand the chemotherapy? What else is there I can do to get stronger and improve my chances at recovery? Does chemotherapy even make sense? What are the alternatives?" Dr. Fernandez-Meier struggles to find the right words, but before she can finish, the patient's husband has already raised another question. The patient is a dental technician, and he's a building engineer; she only wants some answers, and he wants all of them. He is looking for a master plan, Dr. Fernandez-Meier feels.

"Please don't get upset," she tells him, "but the human being is not a machine—it doesn't always allow our plans to be carried out in full."

"I don't understand," he retorts. "You're a trained doctor, surely you must be able to tell me what the best plan is for my wife?"

"Right, but the plan is only for general orientation, it has to be adapted to the individual patient. Let's let your wife ask the questions for a change, and then we can come back to your questions."

If someone's partner gets too involved, it can become all too easy to lose sight of the person for whom your message is actually intended. In this case, the important thing is to keep the actual addressee in mind, and to come back to the initial priorities of the conversation. It is not all that easy to simply ignore one's own state of mind—in this case, the doctor's concern about her mother's illness.

Most misunderstandings during conversations arise due to conflicting roles from a lack of clarity about the role of one's counterpart and/or different, unspoken expectations in the room. As someone communicating bad news, it is beneficial to be aware of and explicitly state one's role ahead of time.

Defining this role can help to establish the necessary amount of emotional and cognitive distance from the content of the message and can be done without losing empathy when delivering the news. Roles may conflict, for example, if the person communicating the news is the doctor, but also the life partner or a close friend of the person receiving the news.

My mother, for example, a former wing assistant at a Berlin hospital, would regularly delegate any conversations about her various illnesses to me—diabetes, arthrosis, asthma, uterine cancer, obesity, high blood pressure, and heart failure—even though I didn't want to take on the task. I felt that I lacked objectivity when speaking with my mother, whom I loved so much, and that this had a negative impact on my medical decisions. Instead, I accompanied her only as a "navigator," leaving the subsequent medical steps at my colleagues' discretion. I refrained from making any decisions, or at least from the vast majority; once or twice I had to stop colleagues, who out of a false understanding of consideration had ordered additional examinations, even though medically speaking there was no additional information to be expected from them.

When the recipients of bad news or their relatives are themselves in a medical profession, some type of conflict is often a given. All too often in these cases, different roles get confused. I recently met the husband—himself an ophthalmologist, but not a cancer doctor—of a patient suffering from an acute case of cancer. Even before we entered the office, the husband was listing all the facts of her case without my asking for them; I could see how concerned he was, and that he was trying to figure out the best way to proceed with operations for his wife. I asked him to hold off with his report for the moment, greeted the patient, and asked if she could describe her difficulties to me. Somehow, both seemed to relax as she began to speak and he was able to focus on his role as her husband. Throughout the conversation, I spoke to the husband as though his wife were one of his patients; I try to address such conflicts head on, showing appreciation and collegial respect, while at the same time making it clear that relatives cannot determine or control medical care. Trust is the foundation for a working doctor–patient relationship—that applies independently of whether the patient or her relatives have a medical background or not.

Time and again, I find that younger doctors in particular avoid conversations in which they have to share difficult news with patients. Often, doctors justify their hesitation by explaining that they lack the sufficient technical skill to give a full picture of the illness, and/or the experience to describe possible treatment options. Over the years, I have heard the same reasoning used in seminars at the Charité Hospital (see more on this in the Appendix) when we call for volunteers to conduct conversations with simulated patients—(lay) actors who act out certain standardized medical histories. Such conversations are a highly effective learning and training method for medical students and doctors, as the patients can give structured feedback on the doctor-patient talk. In the seminars, the urologist declines to speak with an HIV patient, the gynecologist with the relatives of someone who has died in a traffic accident. As most participants quickly realize, however, it is less about the details of the illness than it is about how practically to communicate the news. I also hear regularly from young doctors that they avoid such conversations because they feel they are too far down in the hierarchy, have too little experience, or are afraid of making recommendations that are either wrong or have yet to be fully agreed on. Of course, it is helpful to have a treatment plan at one's disposal, which has been worked out in conjunction with an experienced doctor. As it turns out, however, treatment is not the key issue for this type of conversation, and few, if any details truly need to be communicated. It cannot be repeated often enough: First and foremost, it is about empathy and confronting a difficult situation head on.

I do not mean for empathy to be misunderstood as a sort of unrestricted attention or care; it is absolutely necessary for the person communicating the bad news to maintain some internal distance, so that he does not lose a piece of himself with each additional piece of bad news. This doesn't mean that one should ignore their own feelings; to the contrary, these feelings are important to notice and reflect on, if only to better understand their own reactions and behavior. This knowledge can also improve one's conversational techniques and responses, and help one to cope with grief, compassion, and anger. Without a certain distance, one loses their sense of objectivity, and in doing so truthfulness. One study of English doctors by Lesley Fallowfield—a key figure in research on the doctor–patient relationship—showed dramatic results: When doctors were particularly sympathetic with their patients, it was difficult for them to communicate the true findings of an examination and/or a bad piece of news.

Doctor, Why Am I So Hoarse?

I am drinking coffee with steamed milk and a little nutmeg again—it does me good after difficult operations—dictating the operation report when the telephone rings. My secretary has Professor Steinführer, a colleague, on the line. She asks if I have a moment to speak.

"What can I do for you?" I ask.

"I've been hoarse for 2 weeks—can that be from the new medication they prescribed me?"

"Do you have a cold? Any cough or fever?" I continue, expecting a quick yes, that it's winter and there's a cold going around. "No, I don't have a cough, or a fever for that matter," she replies.

She has just been to the ear, nose, and throat doctor who, after examining her throat with an angled mirror, informed her that her left vocal cord was paralyzed, and that a tumor was one possible cause. I ask her to come to the hospital—around 1 o'clock I have to oversee the end of the state exam I am administering today. She adds that she's hoping to travel to Chemnitz tomorrow with her nephew, to celebrate the holidays with her 89-year-old mother.

She's waiting for me when I get to my office. I feel her throat but don't detect any swollen or suspicious lymph nodes; the neurologic tests taken to this point don't show any irregularities, either. I have her touch her nose with her eyes closed and take several steps—her fine motor skills are also in perfect condition. "I'll be fine through the New Year, don't you think? Should I take cortisone?" asks Professor Steinführer.

I recall from my medical training that, due to its anatomical position, the nerve leading to the vocal cords can sometimes be damaged in thyroid surgery. But she hasn't had any operations. I recommend that she have magnetic resonance imaging (MRI) taken of her throat and brain. Although it is early Friday afternoon, I call and ask a colleague to perform the procedure. He says he will try and promises to call back in a couple of minutes. And it turns out, we are in luck: they schedule an examination 2 hours from now. News of the short-term appointment comes as a relief; my colleague tells me that we will even have the results back today. By 6 P.M. Professor Steinführer is back—the doctor told her to come see me immediately. For a moment, the roles have changed: I am the one receiving, she the one communicating the bad news.

"It looks bad" is the first thing she says as we sit down.

"What do you mean, bad?" I ask.

"Really bad," she replies. The paralysis is caused by a metastatic brain tumor. She's depressed, as am I—we've known each other for years.

"So what happens now?" she asks. I recommend that she be hospitalized and treated with cortisone to reduce any swelling caused by the malignant growth. Cortisone treatment can also counteract the paralysis of the vocal cord, even if only temporarily. "It's crazy," I think, "most women with brain metastases show completely different clinical symptoms, headaches, unsteadiness when walking, or nausea and vomiting."

"Please stay here," I tell her. "Drive to your mother's if you absolutely must, but that is your responsibility. You could suffer an epileptic attack at any minute—I have to tell you that. On Monday I'll request whole-brain radiation treatment. I'm sorry, but it really is serious, Professor Steinführer."

She seems to take it all in stride. She looks up and asks, "I can hope that I won't die too soon, right?"

"I don't know, but I want to be honest with you—this may be your last Christmas with your mother," I tell her.

One night has passed since the bad news. She was able to sleep—she wanted to leave immediately for Chemnitz when her nephew picked her up, but together they decide to remain in Berlin after all. "I'm not afraid, and physically I feel well," she says. I offer for her to stay in the hospital, but she would rather be at home. "What should I look for?" she asks. "Please don't stay at home by yourself," I urge. "My brother is coming in tomorrow morning," she answers, "and my landlord knows about it. The loneliness and uncertainty won't get the best of me." "Is your voice better?" I ask before we hang up. "Not yet!" she replies.

The next morning she writes to me: "Last night was better, so is my voice. Have a great weekend, yours, Prof. Steinführer."

How Do I Start a Conversation When Sharing Bad News?

Proceed gradually, as it were, leaving it to the recipient to decide for herself how much information and explanation she would like to hear, and the pace at which it should be communicated. Never underestimate the patient, however, or any recipient of bad news for that matter. If anything is unclear, ask, leaving space for each answer and reaction. You may also feel your way toward the subject with your own words, asking about the patient's current situation and expectations, her time frame, and whether there is a person she trusts whom she would like to be there. The person's right to "not wanting to know" that I previously mentioned should also be respected, although this shouldn't be taken as a free pass "not to inform." The task can even be delegated to a trusted person—just ask.

What I do tell my patients and their relatives proactively is that I will not lie in the conversation and that telling them the truth is very important to me. Without this attitude, I wouldn't be able to develop patient treatment plans I could fully support.

When breaking bad news, many people are afraid of letting slip the wrong phrase or individual word, and thus focus on speaking in short, simple sentences and clear expressions. What happens if I choose the wrong word, or a linguistic complication crops up? There is no surgeon alive who has never caused some sort of complication during a surgery, for example, damaging the ureter (the narrow duct through which urine passes from the kidney to the bladder) or a section of the intestine, given their complicated anatomical positioning. The trick lies in the ability to recognize the mistake quickly and take any measures necessary to overcome it—in this case, restitching the ureter with surgical thread and inserting a ureteral stent. When sharing bad news, linguistic errors can similarly sneak in that, nevertheless, may have much less of an impact on the relationship than feared and may not stick in people's memories for long.

Difficulties in Understanding

Doctors often encounter patients who seem to be working with completely different information than what their documented medical files would lead one to expect. Some patients, for example, have been told multiple times that they are incurably sick and have experienced numerous relapses—recurrences in their illnesses—yet nevertheless interpret the information in their prognosis differently than one might anticipate. "Doctor, I know that it's serious again," one patient suffering from a severe case of ovarian cancer once said to me. "You can heal me though, right? That's why I'm with you, you're a top specialist." It would have been much easier simply to say yes; the expectation hung thickly in the air between the patient and myself. "No," I replied, truthfully, much to the disappointment of the patient and her husband. I'm a trained doctor, but I'm also an empathetic human being. It always takes a great deal of strength to say this "no" out loud and potentially to bring forth negative feelings. It was the right thing to do, however, and I would do the same today.

Especially in the case of chronic and long-term diseases, I regularly witness how difficult it is for relatives to truly absorb the actual, life-threatening situation. It is as though many are thinking: "It's always been serious or critical, but my wife [mother, sister, etc.] has always gotten through it!" In such cases, I talk about "perpetual death" and "losing one's fear of death."

At one point or another, however, the main subject of the conversation must be brought up. I strongly recommend giving advance warning here: "I'm sorry, but now I have some difficult news for you" might be one way of saying it. A cautious but direct warning, followed by a short pause before the actual news is delivered, is important. It's the same as when someone crashes into your car from behind at a low speed: your chances of survival are better if you see it coming and are buckled up. There can be serious physical consequences even at low speeds, but especially when the accident occurs suddenly, without warning.

The patient also has an unqualified right to not know. For that reason, doctors should never assume that their counterparts will understand and assimilate everything they are hearing, even if it is explained clearly and comprehensibly. When explaining an operation or medical intervention, a doctor should carefully question the patient to find out how much she knows, and above all, what she has understood, so that she can then communicate it to her relatives or those close to her. A patient's understanding of her own illness, treatment, and prognosis may also change over the course of the disease and should be reviewed with every new development.

Sociocultural differences deserve just as much consideration when it comes to problems of comprehension. To avoid misunderstandings with people from other cultural spheres who may have a different approach to information and patient explanations, a short explanation of how these conversations usually proceed may be in order. It can be useful, for example, to begin with a statement such as "generally, we explain everything openly and honestly to patients when the test results have all come back. Do you agree?" As a rule, relatives should not know more than the patient, unless the patient has expressly articulated this wish.

Conversations with people whose language one does not speak present additional challenges. Translators play a crucial role in these situations, acting as a medium between the person who is actually being addressed and the person conveying the news. One should be forewarned that as a form of indirect communication, this configuration is almost certain to make the conversation more difficult. Not only must all the medical information be translated correctly—something one can rarely verify for himself—but the emotional and empathetic dimensions previously discussed must also be taken into consideration. At times, translation's staggered form of communication can create a disconnect between information and emotion—a risk that one should always try to avoid. Conversations in translation also tend to take longer compared to a standard two-person conversation and may suffer from extended, awkward pauses. Once he has finished speaking, the bearer of the message should keep in mind that the translator must also cognitively and emotionally process the information he has just received. Then there is the actual recipient of the news, who also needs time to take in the information and its implications. Even if the conversation will take longer with three than it would with two, it is still important to pause for breath and allow space. This can work by maintaining good eye contact and keeping your body turned toward the other person, even while your message is being translated into the other language. It's not easy and requires patience, but it pays off—for your counterpart, for the conversation, and for you. Proceeding slowly can also uncover any misrepresentations or distortions that may have occurred in translation, or even prevent them from occurring in the first place. Often the shame and fear translators themselves feel, or simply verbal misunderstandings arising from difficulties in comprehension, can lead them to mistranslate what the doctor has said. The emotional level is never lost, however, as this is also communicated nonverbally, through one's body language, gestures, and facial expressions. Although it is of course ideal to work with a professional, medically trained translator, this is rarely a possibility. Often, the translator is a (remote) relative or friend who is not fully comfortable in both languages. In such cases, what I have written about empathy and addressing the emotional level applies even more.

Consider political summits where two heads of state meet who do not share a language. Usually, the translator remains somewhat hidden, sitting off to the side while the two politicians sit across from each other and maintain eye contact. Such an arrangement could also be ideal for a doctor–patient conversation in translation. If this can't happen, at least try and find a position with a direct view toward the intended recipient. Ask beforehand, however, whether such a seating arrangement is acceptable for the person; many people find it irritating to have someone sitting directly behind them. Moreover, pay attention to any conflicting roles that may arise when families are involved. When in doubt, call in a professional translator.

Why Silence Is Sometimes the Best Answer

Invariably, the most important thing is to take one's counterpart into consideration, and to communicate in a way that gives space to both sides. This explains why one should deliberately make a brief pause after delivering bad news. According to one study from the University of Düsseldorf, a doctor interrupts his patients about once every 11–24 seconds. This is understandable—the doctor is involved and engaged and wants to explain. Interrupting also makes the conversation's progression more difficult, however. In general, doctors should speak less and listen more, allowing their patients sufficient space to offer up their own viewpoints and emotional signals, words, and gestures. As doctors, we can and should also receive training in the art of *not* speaking—pauses are some of the most important conversational tactics at our disposal. It's a common mistake: the patient isn't given a moment to think and ceases to be able to absorb information. In many cases, the patient is simply inundated with information. "Here's your diagnosis, prognosis, and a detailed treatment plan—do you agree?" While this pace may help physicians navigate the seemingly simpler and less emotional professional level, it often leaves patients behind. It is a rewarding practice to see how long one can refrain from speaking during a conversation. The goal here is not to absent oneself from the conversation but rather to join in a dialogue—simply without words—by taking on the role of listener and observer.

Various studies have shown that after receiving bad news, it takes patients only a few seconds to pull themselves together somewhat and begin to ask questions. Doctors shouldn't interrupt this silence or try to fill it with statements like, "There's still this or that option for treatment" or "There may also be another possibility." There may only be several seconds separating the bearer of bad news from the recipient, but to many they feel like hours. And that is as it should be; even if a doctor and patient feel close to one another, each occupies a different role in the situation. We must be capable of facing this silence that, by the way, is often more difficult for the person sharing the news than for the one receiving it. The person affected often experiences such pauses as healing and strengthening, and much more effective than any additional commentary.

Try the following experiment yourself: Imagine that you have to tell an important person in your life that their life partner has just been in an accident. Even if it is somewhat uncomfortable for you, please try and say the following sentence out loud: "Dear ..., I have to tell you that your husband/wife was just in a very serious car accident." Now count silently up to 20. Maybe now you have an idea of how difficult it is to hold this silence.

In the Stairwell

She is 31 weeks pregnant with her first child, lying in the neurosurgical intensive care unit. She was able to come to Berlin from central Poland with the help of donated funds; there are metastases in her head, but she still holds out hopes of an operation and recovery. Maya Nowak is only 32 years old and has already received chemotherapy during her pregnancy for metastatic growths in her lungs, liver, and bones. The breast cancer reentered her body and life with unimaginable force—all the doctors agree that an operation makes little sense. Everyone is focused now on saving the life of the child. The mother is emaciated and very weak; she is in unbearable pain due to the bone metastases. Not even morphine works well anymore, but they haven't been able to give her other medication due to her pregnancy. Dr. Jacek Grabowski, born in Wagroweic, Poland, is speaking with the patient and her husband. It's a stroke of luck—he's well-versed in cancer medicine and speaks perfect German and Polish. Without understanding a single word, I can see that it's a difficult conversation.

Speaking in a soft voice, Dr. Grabowski explains that an operation doesn't make sense. It's not easy for him, and he tries to leave her with some hope. He can't bring himself to talk about death right now. Several times over the course of the conversation, he considers revealing the bitter truth that her disease is incurable, and she will soon die. His eyes say what his lips cannot. Afterward, he tells me it simply would have been too much. Having seen their distraught faces myself, I'm sure he's right. He promises to come back the next day. We say goodbye and begin preparing for tomorrow's C-section.

Two days have passed. The child is in the world and doing well; the operation went off without complications: 46 cm and 1640 g are the joyful little baby's first statistics. Yesterday the patient felt better, and Dr. Grabowski was able to speak with her about a living will. Together with her husband, the patient laid out her medical limits. She is still very weak, her movements still slowed by the amount of morphine. The pain has finally subsided, however, and twice a day the child is brought to her to feel the warmth and love of his mother. The silence in the room is broken only by the mother's heavy breathing—her child, on the other hand, breathes easily, seeming to take joy in the air itself. The child's eyes are closed, but you can feel that he is able to see.

The mother lies in bed, the child in an incubator. On the side of the incubator are two small windows closed off by a thin band of rubber, through which one can reach in. The mother strokes her child, first his little hands, then his feet, then his tender head. Her breathing seems to come more easily now, she moves gracefully and shows no sign of physical weakness. With each day that passes, however, the young mother grows weaker and weaker; everything has become difficult for her. She sleeps for longer and longer spells. The grandparents called today; they are too old to make the trip to Berlin.

What is to be done? What are the next steps? Who makes the next move? Who is capable of asking these questions aloud and confronting the difficult answers? I call Dr. Grabowski from a conference in Stuttgart; he's out of the office today. I ask about the patient, and he tells me that all the preparations have been made to take her home today. But how can he tell the woman's parents that their grandchild has just arrived and in a few days they will have to say goodbye to their daughter forever? The doors to the ambulance close, and it drives off.

Several days later, I meet Dr. Grabowski in the stairwell and ask about the Polish patient with metastasized breast cancer. So far so good, it's been more than 4 weeks since the C-section. The mother is spending a lot of time with the child, and the husband and grandparents are trying to live their lives as normally as possible given the circumstances—despite knowing that in the near future, the mother will die.

The Decisive Question

"What are my chances, Doctor?" I hear this question again and again, usually right after bad news has been delivered. It's often the last and sometimes only question at the end of a conversation. But what do patients mean with the word "chance?" Do they mean their chances at recovery, for improvement in their symptoms or in how they feel generally? Without asking, it remains unclear, and the doctor runs the risk of not answering what the patient actually wants to know. When I encounter this question, I often respond with a question of my own: "Could you try and explain what you mean by chances?" After some back and forth, most patients become more concrete, and I can better answer their question.

Doctors and medical personnel such as nurse practitioners and assistants may be most afraid of a more pointed version of this question: "How much longer do I have to live?" This particular question, however, is asked far less often than one might think, even though nearly half of all cases of cancer cannot be cured and conversations about treatment mostly revolve around palliative care. In this case, palliative care means a treatment plan that focuses on containing or alleviating difficulties such as pain or breathing problems. Operations, chemotherapy, or radiation treatment are then used as additional measures to improve the patient's quality of life—not to extend it. The word "palliative" comes from Latin (*pallium,* cloak; *palliare,* to cloak) and means that only the symptoms of an illness can be alleviated, not its root causes.

One study I worked on involved more than 1800 patients from countries across Europe. The results: some 5%–10% of patients did not want any prognosis on their life expectancy. Many wished for general orientation but not a specific forecast, as they were convinced that no one could predict the exact time of death. Nearly everybody surveyed, however, did want precise information about the side effects that cancer treatment would have as well as its impact on their daily lives. They also wanted to hear about alternatives to the doctor's suggested treatment, as well as a second opinion.

As a young student during my internship, one day I accompanied a doctor on his rounds through the surgery wing. While there, he received a call about making a recommendation for postoperative treatment following a cancer operation. The patient in question was recovering in another department; the professor was now supposed to discuss further treatment with her. The initial suspicion of fallopian tube cancer hadn't been corroborated; rather, it seemed it was stomach cancer scattered throughout the peritoneum. We knocked twice and then opened the door to the patient's room—her husband, who was opening a small container of yogurt, dropped it on the bedside table. Quickly setting it upright, he looked around in some confusion for a garbage can to throw away the lid. We took in the situation while making our way over to the 47-year-old patient's bed. The professor introduced himself and me, sat down, and asked the patient, "Do you have a contract out for a building loan?"

"Yes," she replied somewhat vexed.

"In that case you should cancel it, and sooner rather than later," replied the professor.

Years later, I ran into the very same couple at the hospital; recognizing me from a distance, at first the husband looked away. I walked up to them. "Excuse me," I began, "but aren't you the couple with the building loan contract?" They stood there; the husband raised his head and fixed his gaze on me. I was able to shift my glance to his wife. She was doing well, she said, none of the follow-up examinations had shown any recurrence of the cancer. She beamed at me; it felt good to stand in the rays of human warmth.

"And how was it for you then, when the doctor asked you about the contract?" I continued, taking a risk.

"That was some tough stuff," replied the husband.

"It's true," the wife said, "but I was still grateful to the doctor. I don't hold it against him. He was the first person who was honest with me and made it clear how serious my situation was. And we got our papers in order, which was also really important," she added.

Nevertheless, I would recommend seeking out less brusque paths to the truth. In this case, it was precisely the "one decisive question" that was answered forcefully before it was even asked. It's never about a single word or sentence, and even impromptu expressions that are inappropriate can later be corrected or explained. What counts—and stays—however, is one's attitude and the "taste" that a conversation leaves behind. It should be one of clarity and, above all, truth.

My first meeting with a former patient, Gala, illustrates just how widely these situations can vary. Gala was a well-known painter from Tajikistan who had been living in Berlin with her husband and son for several years. Her family came with her to our first meeting during my visiting hours to discuss a treatment plan for her illness. She was my final patient at the end of a long day. Gala was very slender, with an unmistakable but elegant pallor. She had short blonde hair and wore dramatic neon clothing that revealed a great deal of her pretty skin. She wore very dark makeup under her eyes, and her lips were bright red. She wore a light green tie without a dress shirt and was decked out in a burst of green, pink, and yellow that reminded me of the colorful stalls at the bazaar in Marrakech. Despite the fact that it was the end of the day, I was charmed by the skillful arrangement of colors and the hopeful expression on her face. For their part, her husband and son presented a study in contrast—there was no play with colors; both dressed simply in one shade and barely took part in the conversation.

Gala's tumor had returned, I told her finally, and it would never go away again. After a pause that was difficult for us all, she asked, speaking in a soft voice and a thick Russian accent, not how much longer she might have to live but instead "how long do I still have to paint?"

"That depends on the pictures," I replied, "How long do you need to finish one?"

I had never seen one of her paintings. "That depends," she countered. "Sometimes a month, sometimes 3 or 6 months."

"So you see, the real answer is between zero and many."

Everyone—Gala, her husband, and her son—seemed content with the answer. She smiled and continued: "What kind of medical possibilities are there in that case, to help me paint?"

Truthfulness and Trust

Voltaire wrote that "everything you say should be true, but not everything true should be said." This idea plays a key role for me when it comes to delivering bad news. But who really knows what the truth is, anyway? The truth is a sketch of reality or the factual—a mirror image of what occurs. Doctors often feel themselves obligated to tell the truth and to discuss prognoses or potential future scenarios without being certain of the details or what will happen when or in what way. In conversation after conversation with patients and their relatives, I have noticed my own tendency to describe every last possibility, and to allow my own professional knowledge and medical statistics to dictate the conversation.

"Even though today's examination showed no pronounced results, there is over a 90% chance of your cancer recurring within the next 6 months"—this is an everyday statement at the hospital. I have noticed, too, a feeling of relief at listing off negative facets for patients—might this have to do with the fact that we increasingly regard information and patient explanations from a legal perspective?

I have also observed how difficult it is for patients to maintain eye contact with me when I am describing the medical facts of their prognosis. While many appreciate my directness and honesty, many still want to discuss any possibilities that remain. It is also a conversation I support, even if medical statistics speak against the patient's chances of survival. Physicians should never forget that statistics can only provide orientation; they cannot predict individual cases. Most patients are grateful when I bring up others who have continued to live, and live well despite a bad prognosis. To my mind it is perfectly legitimate and natural as humans to seek hope, and the option of helping to decide what can be done actively. Even if a patient's chances of survival are slim, it is still true that she may survive. We are not promising something that is in actual fact an impossibility—we are informing the patient of all her possibilities.

Who really knows the truth, either his own or that of others? It is entirely possible to share our own views with the patient—what we as doctors hold to be the truth—while also accepting the patient's perspective. It is astounding how infrequently patients are consulted for their opinion. Given that there can be no absolute truth where the future accuracy of the prognosis is concerned, a degree of modesty is in order when delivering it. A doctor should not have a guilty conscience because he hasn't told a patient everything as forcefully as he might have. Lies and false promises are another matter, however, and are never appropriate.

Who knows the truth of any given situation? As a strategy in conversation, communicating what one supposes to be the truth while still allowing room for hope isn't contradictory and can absolutely be incorporated into discussions concerning bad news. To do so, however, there must be trust—and patients seem not always to trust their doctors. Trust is a sort of life elixir for the doctor–patient relationship; without it, a resilient and enduring connection becomes impossible. According to one survey of women with ovarian or breast cancer, however, around 30% of respondents thought their doctor had not told them the truth.

Trust and transparency build the foundations for any successful doctor–patient relationship. Truthfulness and effective communication are particularly important when caring for cancer patients. Clinical results and decisions about treatment should be discussed and explained in a way that is easy for patients to understand, while individual pieces of information should be communicated in short, clearly formulated sentences and in measured amounts, so as not to inundate and finally overburden the patient with information. It isn't necessary to fit everything into one conversation. Precision and thoroughness are not always synonymous with truth. In fact, the truth is often overshadowed by all the information—the patient can't see the proverbial forest for the trees.

I regularly meet doctors through our courses who can't understand why certain patients claim to know nothing about a disease they have sometimes had for decades. Although such patients may have been demonstrably told on multiple occasions about the progression of their illness, they continue to insist that no one has explained their illness, or even shared the bad news with them. In order to preempt this sort of back and forth from the outset, I reiterate here that doctors must first and foremost measure themselves against what the patient has actually understood of what has been said.

What might the reasons be for such an "informational gap?" We could point to any number of explanations without arriving at a final, evidence-based conclusion. Such behavior might be a cry for help—a wish for a closer relationship with the doctor to help confront one's own fears, for example. Perhaps the patient—be it for reasons stemming from her childhood, social environment, current state of health, or a crippling sense of fear and grief—was initially unable to comprehend and accept bad or, what was for her, confusing news. While this topic has generated great interest, academic research has not settled on any real answers. This leads me back to my earlier statement that a person conveying bad news should measure themselves by what stays with the recipient on a lasting basis. In this case, it can also help for a doctor to follow up, making sure that he himself has fully grasped what the news means for his patient and that communication has stayed effective throughout the interaction.

A patient should be able to trust implicitly in the truthfulness of her doctor's answers; any feelings to the contrary should be brought up immediately. A relationship on even footing means that mature patients should play an active role in the conversation. It is particularly important that aside from factual information, the person sharing the bad news communicates respect, esteem, honesty, and a willingness to help with their words; this general attitude should be a guiding star for the conversation. Then, what was a one-sided speech becomes a shared conversation.

Repeat the following four words out loud: respect, esteem, honesty, support. Try reciting these words when preparing for a difficult conversation as a sort of mental and emotional preparation—see what it can do for you.

Allowing Space for Theories of Illness and Speaking with Each Other

Soon after a person receives bad news, the question inevitably occurs: Why did this happen to me of all people? This question is not irrational, in fact it's completely understandable. Moreover, it isn't only the patient who should ask this question, but their entire social network. Engaging with this question can help us to better understand various reactions and develop different approaches to both internal and external conflicts. In this case, too, the same principle applies for doctors: Observe and describe, don't assess.

At one point or another, nearly every patient develops their own subjective theory or theories about their illness. Also called lay concepts, these theories are a type of explanatory model that patients create themselves in order to account for the origin of various illnesses. Discrepancies between a doctor's medical explanations and those of the patient are considered a leading cause of noncompliance, or when a patient fails to follow the doctor's recommendations for treatment. Familiarizing oneself with a patient's subjective theories of illness can help tremendously in better understanding potential biases or doubts about certain types of treatment. Patients often develop these theories when first beginning to cope with their illness. While the models may seem both logical and rational to the patient, they generally remain incomprehensible to doctors and—what is more problematic—often contradict medical explanations for the causes of whichever diseases are under discussion. In such cases, mutual trust—a factor I have repeatedly highlighted as the basis for a functional doctor–patient relationship—either suffers from this disparity or cannot be built in the first place.

One study conducted by my working group surveyed 1,800 women with ovarian cancer from different countries about their lay concepts of etiology—how, in other words, the patients accounted for the origin of their disease. Among the causes, patients listed personal stress, genetic disposition, work stress, poor nutrition, viral infection, environmental pollution, or nicotine. Some women attributed the emergence of their cancer to hormonal influence; other reasons included radioactivity, sexual assault, poisoned food, groin operations, and homesickness. Another study by the same working group showed similar results for patients with breast cancer: stress was frequently listed as a cause. At first glance, a very vague image emerges for doctors. It is an image, however, as varied as life itself, and even from a medical standpoint we can't always say for sure what the causes of an illness are, as much as we would like to, and continue to pursue research to that end.

A doctor can exert an influence on a patient's subjective theories of his illness; to do so the doctor must be aware of these theories to begin with. Doctors rarely consult their patients about these theories explicitly; the patient rarely dares to utter them. If these lay concepts are not discussed openly with the doctor, however, there is a danger that they can become the patient's truth, an incontrovertible certainty on his part. Medical or natural scientific arguments can rarely accomplish anything in these cases; on the contrary, they may even confirm the patient's reasoning in his own mind. This results in uncertainty for the doctor as well as the patient.

To give just one example from my own clinical experience, as a young doctor I once had to recommend chemotherapy to a 45-year-old patient after an operation. I additionally wanted to encourage her to take part in a clinical study as an alternative form of treatment. The study featured three different treatment protocols:

1. Infusions with medication A and medication B
2. Infusions with medication A and medication C
3. Infusion with medication A and tablets with medication D

Medication A was the control treatment method—in principle, the other medications were also effective and already available individually. For the study, the medications were to be administered in combination, however, in the hopes that patients would show less resistance. I gave the patient an exhaustive rundown of all the potential effects and side effects, which did not differ greatly from one another. After I had spoken for about half an hour, the patient asked whether she couldn't choose which of the protocols she was given. I explained that it wasn't permitted in a "randomized study," that the treatments were assigned randomly, and she would be given 1, 2, or 3 without my being able to influence the process.

"Well that's a shame," she answered, crestfallen. "I could do treatments 1 or 2 but not number 3, so I can't take part in your study!"

While I didn't understand and was somewhat disappointed, I also respected her decision. "Why would you accept treatment plans 1 and 2, but not 3?" I asked in an effort to understand her thinking. "After all, all the protocols are based on the same standard medication."

Her reply: "About 4 weeks ago I was in Istanbul and caught a serious gastrointestinal infection from a public toilet. A few days later, I was diagnosed with ovarian cancer. Aside from the peritoneum, the cancer also attacked parts of my intestine."

"And what does that have to do with not taking part in the study?" I continued.

"Don't you see, Doctor? My intestinal infection caused the cancer, so anything that might affect my gastrointestinal tract won't help me recover. That's why I decided not to take any more tablets, so there's no way I could agree to the third treatment plan in the study."

I tried to explain everything to her again from a medical perspective, but I wasn't able to convince her to take part in the study. Today, I realize that in the moment I should have allowed more time to explain and not applied pressure.

Lay hypotheses can provide doctors with insight into why a patient might think that a disease has befallen them. Subjective explanations give patients an initial route to keep living in a way they see fit and to take active countermeasures. Doctors should ask patients explicitly about any ideas they may have regarding the cause of their illness in order to counteract the influence of any false theories but also to allow for improved collaboration. Comprehensive information and explanations are considered central reasons why patients agree to proposed treatment options; it stands to reason that doctor–patient conversations should be given clearer definition. Otherwise, one deprives patients of the chance to weigh various theories about their illness and actively contribute toward its treatment.

The Sad Message about Mamed

My father-in-law comes from Iran; in his time, he was forced to leave his beloved homeland due to his political resistance to the Shah. A great deal has changed over the years in his life abroad. His mom-and-pop store in Berlin's neighborhood of Neukölln became known throughout the city as one of the first of its kind, selling everything from rolls to pocket warmers. Living abroad has also changed his relationship to his siblings, however. For her part, although my wife was born in Berlin, she's always had a strong desire to learn more about her parent's homeland and her own roots—a desire that eventually led her to search for relatives on the Internet.

When she finally did succeed in locating her extended family in the virtual world, she was completely absorbed in the photographs, gladly welcoming each of her relatives into her life. One day she came across an article written in Farsi, the modern form of Persian. It was only upon reading it for a second time that she realized her uncle, her father's elder brother, had died. Here she had been looking for good news about her long lost family and wound up with tragic news about her uncle. How could she bring herself to tell her father? She called her sister first, then her mother. Neither was willing to tell my father-in-law the news of his elder brother's death. My wife looked up at me with her dark eyes, and I knew: it would have to be me.

We picked up my wife's sister in the car and drove out to Rudow in the south of Berlin, where their parents have lived for over 30 years. My father-in-law didn't know we were coming; otherwise, he would have been out in the street, waiting for us. We rang, and my mother-in-law answered. She knew what was happening and followed me inside with her two daughters. My father-in-law could tell that something wasn't right, I could feel it. "I have to tell you something," I began. "Your brother, Mohamed, has died." His eyes opened wide and his mouth fell open. "Mohamed? Who's Mohamed?" he asked. "Mohamed, your brother!" The other three couldn't bring themselves to speak.

"Tell me Jalid, what happened, who died? Do you mean Mamed?" "Yes," I replied, "Mamed!" My father-in-law fell to the ground and began crying. Everyone crowded around to hold him, comforting him greatly.

I asked later if he had a negative memory of the moment when I said the wrong name. "No, Jalid, it wasn't bad at all. I could see from the look in your eyes that you had a sad truth to tell me. I'd actually forgotten that you said the wrong name. What I haven't forgotten is that you took the responsibility to deliver the sad news personally."

THE MESSAGE

I have to tell him,
But how?
Is it better to say nothing?
But can I do that,
Simply keep quiet about the terrible news?
Yet the truth must come out,
It came looking for me to speak it.
But why me?
I accept the burden,
But how to do it?
I will do it for him,
But do I have the strength?
And did the truth ever ask him?
Not a single word,
My eyes and the silence will do it,
The awful news has been passed on,
But our hands will not come apart,
They are joined forever.

JALID SEHOULI

The Bigger Picture: Turning Relatives into Allies

At first glance, it seems better for patients not to face truly difficult conversations on their own but to have someone they feel close to with them. It can help the patient to have somebody with whom she can process the conversation afterward; a third person may also hear and understand more because he isn't as emotionally impacted as the patient herself. What's more, later on the patient doesn't have to recall a conversation she may only partially remember on her own.

All of these reasons would appear to make the idea of someone accompanying the patient an obvious choice. Most would agree without thinking twice, and it does indeed have its advantages. Although it also has disadvantages—the presence of another person receiving the news, for example, is sure to divide the doctor's attention. That means that the patient will no longer receive uninterrupted eye contact or constant attention for any feelings that might arise. Furthermore, the third person in the room may also be disturbed by the news—maybe even more than the intended recipient—and react in unexpected ways. In that case, the doctor or, even worse, the patient may first have to care for the companion.

Questions and answers will also vary. Patients will primarily be concerned with what they can continue to count on and the uncertainties of living with their illness, whether that involves symptoms or a potential loss of bodily functions and diminished sense of self-worth. For relatives or companions, however, it is largely thoughts about the consequences that point to unnerving questions.

Consider this example: A patient has just learned over the course of a conversation that she has breast cancer and disseminated (spreading) lung metastases; she wonders how she will be able to withstand the pain and other forms of suffering. She is also asking herself "the one question" we mentioned previously: *How much longer do I have to live?* For his part, the husband asks himself how he is supposed to manage with three small children once his wife is gone. It is completely natural that each person would think first about the consequences for their own life. But, for example, when the husband then asks the doctor "What does that mean concretely for me?" it can trigger a feeling of great disappointment and sense of abandonment in the wife, maybe even deep anger.

We cannot assume that a patient's relatives will naturally provide a support system, but must instead keep in mind that relatives are often greatly affected themselves and may even be doing worse than the patient herself. Relatives and friends are also involved in the bad news in a direct, immediate sense, and rarely have an opportunity to retreat or set their own boundaries. If a couple has a healthy relationship that is marked by closeness and solidarity, a patient's partner will share in her pain. If this is not the case, however, old, unhealthy patterns of guilt or rage or fears of dependency can surface, posing an additional burden. In either case and for whatever reason, in a group setting, the same questions will be either not asked or posed differently than they would be in a one-on-one conversation. For that reason, it's helpful to check in ahead of time about whether a patient would like someone else to be present and, if the conversation does only take place between the patient and doctor, to make sure that a third person is either available or close by in order to "cushion" the blow. The goal here is to win over relatives as allies.

Although most of a patient's relatives will want to help, many will not be sure about the best way to do so. Moreover, a majority of relatives will themselves be in need of psychological or social support, and doctors should also be able to make suggestions in this regard.

Stressful situations can easily lead to conflicts within families, in which case including family members may not only be unhelpful but may even make things more difficult for the patient. It is better to consult with the patient first—with only the two of you present in the room—about whether he or she would like family to be present.

I am meeting with a 44-year-old patient I operated on several weeks ago for an intestinal obstruction. She's doing much better but is having problems eating and drinking again. She can only eat a small amount before getting nauseous, and her bowels are sluggish. The obstruction cropped up shortly after the patient completed chemotherapy: unfortunately, the peritoneum—the membrane lining the abdominal cavity and covering the abdominal organs—showed extensive damage. The patient is willing to do anything to regain her health and finally overcome the cancer, which has now broken out again after her first diagnosis 2 years ago. "I have to get better," she says.

"How are your parents?" I ask.

"They're doing alright overall, thanks for asking," she replies.

"Have you told them yet that you have a severe case of cancer?" I persist. Several months ago, we discussed broaching the subject with her parents.

"No," she answers, "I can't; they would be ostracized."

"Ostracized?" I can hardly believe what I've heard.

"Yes, ostracized. They live in a very small village; that's how it is there. Just yesterday when I told my mother that I was in the hospital for a harmless gastrointestinal issue, she replied that I was to blame because I overdid it with my eating and all the diets. She always blames me; that's how it has always been. That's why I have to beat the cancer, even if the chances of healing are small. I just can't tell my mother."

I try again to persuade her to tell her parents. The people who you love and know you well, whom you are closely connected to also have a right to know the truth, I tell her. And it might bring some relief to finally be free of her secret—even if it is not as easy to be free of the illness. "All the energy you spend on concealing the disease and the truth, you could use it for other things," I add. She gives me a sad look, then forces a smile and says goodbye; she has another important medical exam to get to.

It is extremely difficult as doctors to have a treatment suggestion that applies to every situation always at the ready. We can also deceive ourselves in this regard—at the end of the day, it is the patient who decides. It is her responsibility to decide who should be told when, and how. The doctor can help the patient to treat this decision and responsibility deliberately, however, and share valuable previous experiences with other patients in similar situations. By the same token, doctors should never inform or instruct the patient's relatives or friends without the patient's consent, even if this is well intended.

"We can't change the direction of the wind, but we can adjust the sails." This quote from Aristotle Onassis serves as a guiding light that I always try to remember when these types of situations come up. Above all, it helps me to keep my own attitude and interests in check vis-à-vis the patients. Simply because I am the doctor treating the patient doesn't mean I decide every step of the treatment or conversation. The fact that patients regularly consult anonymous sources for more information directly after—or in many cases, before—receiving bad news is a particularly sensitive point for many doctors and therapists. Various studies have shown that over 70% of patients either use the Internet or seek a second medical opinion. Doctors shouldn't take offense at a patient seeking orientation and information or interpret this as a doubt in their medical ability, however, but rather view it as a constructive approach to the bad news and/or illness. Affected patients often greatly appreciate concrete forms of assistance from doctors, such as website addresses or informational materials, even if they are not discussed in depth during the conversation. It similarly makes sense to list options for a second opinion straightaway, without the patient having to ask. (It can be difficult for a patient to overcome her doubts in this regard.) According to one study we conducted at the Charité, more than 90% of patients with breast cancer wanted more information about such options, but only a quarter had any.

By the end of the conversation, it is worthwhile to turn toward what happens "afterward." Ideally, one has already assembled some information and possibilities or has a standard set of suggestions on hand. What type of life situation is the patient—the person—returning to? What is her environment? Who is there to help? What personal resources and forms of assistance might help the patient deal with the news? An awareness of these possibilities can also reduce stress for the person conveying the bad news, who is often focused only on the conversation and may feel like he is the only source of support available. Doctors tend to take all the burden on their own shoulders—an enterprise that is doomed from the start.

What human, social, or technical resources are at the patient's immediate disposal? I have already mentioned relatives and people close to the patient, as well as places where the patient can turn for a second and even third opinion. In some cases, it may even be possible to arrange for dedicated care from the hospital or a public social service.

What Helps People to Assimilate Bad News?

I recently met a patient with whom I am very close, who had been through an operation and a difficult chemotherapy treatment since we last spoke. She looked elegant; she had regained all her hair and that day had chosen blue as a fashion statement—even her glasses were sky blue. Over the course of our conversation, I asked about the worst news she had ever received. "My cancer diagnosis," she replied, as if she had been awaiting my question for some time.

"And what helped you to process it?" I asked.

"My children, and tennis."

Her children I could understand, but tennis? "Do you play much tennis yourself?" I continued.

"No, but I teach physical education, and I love to watch. During my illness I didn't want to watch the news or cheesy films. Tennis, on the other hand, is simply about winning or losing. A lot like my cancer diagnosis I thought, when I first found out—that was also about whether I would be able to win or would lose. So watching helped—I especially enjoyed seeing people win. Watching tennis was also a moment when I could be alone; initially I needed to be alone to make sense of my own path. Not wanting to miss any games provided an excuse to take some distance from the well-intentioned but generally frustrating advice I was receiving."

As this anecdote shows, there is no single recipe for how best to deal with bad news; the coping mechanisms a person may have picked up or been taught during early childhood or adolescence are far too varied. It is worthwhile to be aware of such mechanisms, however: Is it human interaction that will help the most? Movement through sports? Painting, pottery, or writing? Doctors can only act as spotters throughout this process, helping the patient discover what is most likely to be of service to them in this regard. Experience shows, however, that when people find themselves in an existential life situation, most know exactly what is best for them—in that much we can trust.

It is also important to get an idea of how resilient the patient is—if possible *before* conducting a difficult conversation. The term *resilience* (from the Latin *resilire*, to rebound or bounce back) originates in research on physical materials and describes highly elastic materials that can return to their original form after being misshapen. Over time, the ability to adapt without buckling or warping permanently came to be applied to peoples' defense mechanisms. In this sense then, resilience means an ability to handle life crises without losing the courage to go on living or collapsing under the strain. This psychic capacity to resist depends first and foremost on an affected person's ability to mobilize personal and/or social resources in grappling with the crisis. In principle, everyone is inclined to withstand a crisis—it is simply that some have greater potential to resist, others less.

For years, science has explored which factors encourage or impair resilience, without, however, finding answers to all the questions. While one's childhood and social contacts seem to play essential roles, support, affirmation, reliability, space, trust, and confidence are also discussed as crucial aspects in academic literature.

In general, resilient people seem to possess a greater awareness of their personal strengths and what they are capable of actively pursuing than people with less resilience. Further, they tend to strike a fundamentally positive or at least discerning attitude toward difficult life situations, allowing them to readily interpret a crisis as a challenge and opportunity for personal growth, and to break out of the role of the victim with greater ease.

An awareness of one's own resilience, then, can help people process bad news. For the bearer of bad news, this means making the patient, or recipient of the bad news, aware of their options. Resilience is also an important quality in people who communicate bad news on a professional basis, as it allows them to detach from emotionally difficult situations and subsequently to recuperate. In this regard, one might ask questions like: How can I improve my resilience in different areas of my life? What has supported my resilience or ability to resist in the past?

Bad news often plunges recipients into a deep bout of mourning, at times even causing them to temporarily lose their bearings. Nevertheless, as the person sharing the news, one should try and help a patient take action, thereby helping the patient regain the feeling that he or she can in some way control or influence their situation. This might take the form of scheduling a follow-up appointment or providing a referral, for example, for another professional expert. The patient has their own ideas about what might help, or the type of support they are looking for.

Possible questions here might include: "How can I best support you now? What do you need help with? Can I contact anyone for you? How are you planning to get home? Is there someone to pick you up? What are you expecting when you go back home/to work?" Asking questions about the potential effects of the bad news on the patient's family, friends, or future prospects may also help the patient prioritize what is most important to him.

Once a doctor has shared a bad diagnosis in conversation, it is important that he or she create sufficient space in what follows by regularly allowing room for pause and delving into whatever feelings he or she perceives in the patient. One might say, for example, "This is very difficult for you right now," then pause before continuing. In every feedback session, simulation patients single out pauses as some of the most important—and helpful—moments in the conversation.

In contrast, the sentence "I realize how difficult this must be for you" almost always elicits negative reactions among simulation patients. Most patients take it to be a superficial cliché that offers small comfort; it may even make people angry. "What exactly do you know about what this means for me and my life, as a doctor, with your social position and your health! You have no idea what this means for me!" as one simulation patient put it in a feedback session, when asked about her unspoken thoughts.

In another simulated conversation, we imagined the following situation: A 78-year-old patient has just found out that she has a highly aggressive form of leukemia in its terminal phase. She gasps audibly and looks out past the open door. "Doctor, I'm scared!" she says. In the simulation, the doctor's response concentrated entirely on the word "scared." "Scared? You don't need to be scared," the doctor replied without asking any follow-up questions. "There are any number of treatment possibilities available." In the follow-up conversation, the simulation patient revealed that the doctor's response hadn't even registered as she had been overwhelmed by a feeling of fate dealing her an unfair hand and thoughts about her sick husband. What, she immediately asked herself, would become of him if she were to die? In the moment, the fear that her husband would not receive care surpassed even the fear of her own death. The doctor did not ask what the patient was scared of but rather interpreted this for her needs, jumping straightaway into a discussion of possible treatments and preventing the patient's concerns about her cherished husband from emerging in the first place. In this case, questions like "Scared of what?" or "What are you worrying about right now?" could have helped the patient to make her fears somewhat more concrete by naming them. It would then have been easier to handle, even to assuage them.

Some years ago while working as a young assistant medical director, I had to share some bad test results from an interim assessment with a 24-year-old patient. The patient had just undergone a third round of chemotherapy for a case of advanced cervical cancer that had already been heavily treated; her husband was a professional soccer player, who could rarely come to her appointments. The patient had placed great hopes in the demanding treatment—she was committed to doing everything she could to watch her 3-year-old child grow up. Accompanied by a young doctor, I went up to her room where I found her receiving a visit from her mother. The neighboring patient wasn't doing well either, so I asked if, despite some swelling in her right leg, the patient would come with us into the conference room. Her eyes opened wide, but she forced a smile in spite of the fear I could see in her expression. "Yes!" She answered in a loud voice.

It was a 50-foot walk over to the conference room—the entire way there I couldn't think of a single thing to say. The young doctor knew that in a few moments we would have to deliver the bad news. She had a good relationship with the patient; they shared a similar taste in music, and she often came in at the end of her night shift to ask about the young woman with terminal cervical cancer. When we finally arrived, I opened the door without knocking, only to find the room was occupied—I could sense that here, too, there was no good news to be had. We went into the neighboring examination room, which was considerably smaller and unfortunately had no windows, even though none of this occurred to me at the time. One of the nurses slipped into the room behind us.

Only the patient and I sat down—the mother, the nurse, and the young doctor remained standing, holding onto the shoulders and hands of the patient. She looked at me steadily and asked: "Well, what are the results? Everything's smaller, right? Tell me!" Hoping no one would notice, I drew a deep breath. "Unfortunately, I have something else to tell you." I forced myself to pause briefly. "After three cycles of chemotherapy, the test results aren't good." I paused again. "I'm sorry, but the cervical cancer has grown." "Whaaaaat?" The patient screamed. Then came the question: "Does this mean I have to die now?"

I bit my tongue. I didn't want to answer, didn't want to say that we all have to die at some point, that it's our fate and life isn't always fair. I bit down on my tongue harder and harder. Everyone was crying: the patient, her mother, the nurse, and even the young doctor. I felt badly—I was sad, but I wasn't crying along with them. Even though I was only communicating the bad news, somehow I felt responsible, like I had caused the disease. I had been the one to suggest the most recent treatment, hoping along with the patient that things might improve, even though the chances were slight. She had struggled through the treatment despite all the side effects and symptoms from the cancer itself, and now she had come for her reward. Had I promised her too much? Had I robbed her of what valuable time remained? The situation was unbearable. I did feel capable of touching her, because I had never touched her before—our meetings had always revolved around the next treatment, and we had shaken hands only a few times. Sometimes fear can put an unwelcome distance between people. The dull pain in my tongue slowly resided as I counted off the seconds in my mind, waiting for the patient's initial reaction to subside. It felt like an eternity, during which I could barely look her in the eye. The rest stood clustered around the patient, holding her and weeping. Then came the reaction I was hoping for.

"And what now?"

"Do you want to continue talking now or at a later point?" I asked.

"Now!" she replied, "but everyone else please leave the room."

"Everyone?" I asked.

"Everyone, except for you!"

The mother, nurse, and young doctor all deferred to the patient, casting a short sad look back as they left the examination room. Once we were alone, I turned to her and asked: "Why did you want everyone to leave the room? They're very concerned about you, and everyone just took a part in hearing the bad news, even the young doctor who's always asking about you."

"That's true," she replied, "but they also cried just like me. That's all well and good, but they can't do anything else. Please tell me, what are my options now?"

The way in which the young woman reacted to what was, for her, a catastrophic diagnosis was indeed unusual, but not completely atypical. There is no prescribed course of events for these sorts of situations, and one can't rely on a set pattern of reactions. One also doesn't need to fear patients becoming physically aggressive upon receiving bad news; most feel somewhat paralyzed, or like the floor has just dropped out from under them. Only once in the course of my entire professional career have I witnessed a patient who stood up after hearing her diagnosis and beat on the door, before collapsing and beginning to cry. One constantly reads stories in the press about patients attacking doctors later on—days, maybe weeks after a diagnosis. According to one study from Munich's Technical University, one out of every four family doctors reports having been attacked at least once by a patient over the course of his career. To this day, however, the actual reasons for these attacks have not received sufficient explanation. Did it involve difficulties in communication or overcoming the disease, or maybe suspected errors in treatment?

Upon hearing bad news, patients and their relatives may, however, react physically. Over the course of my career, I've witnessed people experience sudden bouts of pain, even slight fainting fits. The latter were not truly dangerous; in general, one should try to stay calm and make sure that the person does not hurt themselves falling. If the patient does fall, lay them flat on the floor and elevate their legs; usually a "vasovagal syncope" is the cause. In syncope, the brain temporarily receives less blood than normal, triggering a rapidly occurring and short-term loss of consciousness that is generally accompanied by losing control of their posture. Causes include certain triggers such as psychic stress, but also cold or pain. Both times this has occurred over the course of my professional life, we were able to continue our conversation at the patients' request once they came back to themselves, and both sides left with a good feeling.

I am struck time and again in my observations by the tension evident in doctor-patient conversations, despite their routine nature. Even doctors who have been trained and instructed to speak in short, simple sentences regularly use unclear formulations and numerous technical terms, which the patient can't understand but rarely trusts himself or herself to ask about. Most patients simply let the doctor continue to speak, in the hopes that they will somehow grasp the essential elements.

I remember a long-term patient who came in once for a follow-up examination. She had lived through a number of heavy blows in her life: her husband died unexpectedly following an operation, her favorite aunt died of a heart attack, then her granddaughter died in a plane crash. Fifteen years before, she developed a case of breast cancer, followed by ovarian cancer 5 years ago. Then, unexpectedly after such a long time, she had a relapse. If such relapses—also called recurrences—do occur, they normally do so within 5 years, but now the cancer had attacked her lungs and liver. For the moment, she was being treated with antibodies and was tolerating it well: she showed no hair loss and normal blood values, only her physical weakness made things more difficult. Happily, a bone analysis had revealed no metastases; even though this had no direct bearing on what was otherwise a very serious prognosis, we were happy about the results.

I asked her about the worst news she had ever received in her lifetime—if it were possible to choose, that is. We had known each other for such a long time that I took the liberty to pursue my curiosity. "The death of my husband!" She replied immediately.

"Why?" I asked.

"Because I was so close to him and his death came totally unexpectedly: a call in the middle of the night from a young doctor. He said he was sorry, and that I could choose whether I wanted to go in straight away to see my dead husband or preferred to wait until tomorrow. I felt paralyzed, in shock, but I took a taxi straight to the hospital. I walked up to his hospital wing and found my husband lying there, dead. The neighboring patient was also really sick and probably somewhat confused—his bed was separated by a folding screen. I could barely speak, and the young doctor started to cry when he saw me. I couldn't bring myself to cry."

"How did it make you feel when the young doctor started to cry?" I asked.

"I was somewhat touched, but I was more furious."

"Why furious?" I wanted to know.

"Because I needed help myself, but no one was asking me how I would get home or how I would get through that night. The young doctor gave me my husband's belongings and asked if I would agree to an autopsy. 'Yes,' I replied, without meaning it. I went home and grew angrier and angrier. I couldn't bring myself to say goodbye to my husband, but I couldn't bring myself to say that at the hospital, either. I was simply too weak. My rage blocked my grief."

Compassionate relationships are not only important for healthy people; they are also important for people who are incurably sick. Anyone will understand this thought; it may even sound banal to some. On three separate occasions, for example, I have known patients who suffered from incurable forms of cancer for years before finally marrying on the day they passed away. To this day, the story of a 33-year-old post office employee with a case of breast cancer and liver and lung metastases still touches me. Time and again the patient insisted to her family and close friends that she would only stand in front of the altar with a full head of hair, even though she had to heal beforehand and the doctors had warned her repeatedly that her wish would be extremely difficult to fulfill. As a young doctor, I listened closely to the conversations among the head doctors, noting how they consistently avoided telling her the truth directly, encouraging her dream instead.

"Of course we'll all be singing in the choir at the wedding," the head doctor said during one visit.

In the end, suffering from a case of jaundice after her liver gave out and could no longer process toxins, and speaking only with great difficulty despite the assistance of an oxygen tank due to the metastases in her lungs, the patient asked for a wedding to be arranged in the hospital ward. It was her final wish; the most important thing was to live that moment before saying goodbye.

From the perspective of a patient and her relatives, such final goals can help us learn to let go. This moment of release continues to impress me—it is sad, yet it also has a grandeur, something sublime about it.

I write this upon returning from the funeral of a patient who recently died after living with ovarian cancer for years—an extraordinary woman. She stayed positive throughout innumerable setbacks, organizing remarkable private art shows at her home in Potsdam and acting in informational films for people affected by cancer and their relatives. She was alert, attentive, and wise, and I always looked forward to my meetings with her, which were more often about life itself and its possibilities than they were medical results.

No one would have noticed her severe cancer or signs of treatment just by looking. She always knew what she wanted and what she didn't. Even in the final days, when she told me that she no longer wanted to receive treatment for the growing cancer, she maintained that all the decisions she had made regarding her treatment had been right for her. She had experienced and accomplished wonderful things, now she simply wanted to sleep. She asked her daughter to return from a vacation in Crete and accompany her to the hospital in Berlin. Her daughter arrived, and a few hours later my patient fell asleep forever.

The Leap

I met with an old friend who lost her 35-year-old son several months ago. At 16 years old he was at the top of his class, but gradually he began to change; it became increasingly difficult for him to cope day to day, and he was plagued by a constant restlessness. Dissatisfied with his own life, he read day and night about life after death. My friend couldn't get through to him, nor could anyone else for that matter. The doctors diagnosed him with schizophrenia and prescribed powerful medication. Over the years, he attempted to take his own life a total of four times by jumping out of windows. His most recent jump, from the second story of his apartment, had been particularly serious; he broke so many bones that he could no longer walk and was bound to a wheelchair. Then, he jumped again.

He was living in Stuttgart at the time, his father in Osnabrück and my friend in Berlin. The parents had divorced years ago; now their son had been found on the street at 6 A.M., dead after his final jump. At first, relatives in Stuttgart were too afraid to tell my friend directly and tried her partner. He was in a meeting, however, and couldn't be reached; they had to tell the mother after all. Although she had been expecting such a call for a long time, when she got the news she couldn't breathe. She hung up without saying a word, then called her partner. "Angelo, I have to go to Stuttgart immediately, my son just jumped again."

"Of course, of course, I'll arrange a flight right away and be over," he replied. After several minutes, however, he began to feel that there was something different about this time. He called back. "You didn't say anything about the hospital, where is he now?" he asked.

"Angelo, he jumped for the last time," came the reply.

They had been planning to travel to Sicily the next day; now they had to repack, removing their evening wear and summer clothing and leaving the suitcases half-empty.

"Would it have been better if your relatives had been able to get in touch with your partner and he had told you the news?" I asked her.

"No, I was grateful to hear about it directly—he's my son after all, and I want to be the first one to find out the truth."

"And what helped you get through it?" I continued.

"Crying, my friends' support, and writing."

"Writing?"

"Yes, writing," she replied. She reached into her bag to take out a small note from her wallet and handed it to me. I unfolded the blue sheet and read the title: "The Leap." I read the first sentence: "I'm crying out of helplessness and screaming out of anger—and I'm praying in the hope that I will not have to keep crying from anger and helplessness."

Writing can help us to articulate our feelings, to make them visible. In the case of creative writing, it is more about a process of self-reflection, a sort of dialogue with oneself, than it is the finished product. A little over a year ago, we began to offer our cancer patients at the Charité hospital and their relatives the chance to do creative writing, and the response has been tremendous.

Writing one's memoirs or keeping a diary are other forms of creative writing, while professionally led therapeutic writing sessions intended to help participants' overcome difficult or existential news on a lasting basis can also help tremendously. These methods should not be seen as opposing but rather complementing other approaches that may involve psychology or painting, art, or movement therapy. They are another opportunity to enter a one-on-one dialogue with people.

Learning from Life Experience

I am on one of my visits to the outpatient clinic; I generally come once a week to see how the daily work is proceeding. *Visit* comes from the Latin (*visitare*), which translates literally as "go to see." I enjoy my visits to patients, although I often feel more like the host than a guest.

Seven women are currently receiving their chemotherapy treatment; the medication drips down from the infusion pumps slowly into their veins, fighting the cancer. It is quiet in the room, although the silence is constantly interrupted by alarms signaling an empty infusion bottle. The women lie in dark-colored armchairs and occupy themselves in different ways. One appears to be listening to music, another is eating fruit, a third reads a Swedish crime novel, while a fourth crochets blue stockings. I take a seat to ask each patient how she is doing and to listen to their problems. I am struck by the general lack of complaints, despite the aggressive medication being administered. A peaceful kind of intimacy hangs in the air, prompting further questions: "What helped when you first found out that you had cancer?"

A 58-year-old patient with a light accent is first to answer: "My family and my experience."

"What experience?" I ask.

"My life experience," she replies. "As a young girl in Poland I lived through a famine. Later I came here to Germany, where I learned the language. That was very difficult—I didn't have any friends, and there was nobody to help me. But I boxed my way through again. That's how I know that I will make it, despite my cancer."

"When did you become aware of your strength?" I ask.

"At first I was really shaken when the doctors told me 3 years ago that I had ovarian cancer, and made it clear to me that I was in the end stages and there were no chances for recovery. I didn't leave my apartment for 3 days and didn't speak with anyone—I had to be alone. I don't even remember the first day. The second day was full of grief. Then, on the third day, I went out onto my balcony and began to water my flowers and thought back on all the difficult moments I had lived through." She beams at me as though she has just won the lottery.

To her right lies a patient who is around 35 years old. She lays her book down and says, "I helped myself, nobody else. When the doctor gave me the bad news, I sat down in the first restaurant I could find and ordered the most expensive meal they had. I still remember exactly what it was: a saddle of venison with fresh chanterelle mushrooms and blueberries, with a wild strawberry mousse for dessert. Afterward, sitting there, I remember taking a long look at the small, gold baroque hand mirror I had inherited from my grandmother, and which I always keep with me. "Do you want to live, or to die?" I whispered—I didn't want to disturb the neighboring tables. At that moment the waiter arrived, an attractive, tall, and slender man. "Would you like anything else?" he asked in a friendly voice. "Yes," I answered, "I'd like to live, please."

The patient sitting across from me is next to speak. She wears a head scarf—she comes from Tunisia and speaks a wonderful German with French undertones. "God helped me greatly. He heard my doubts and turned them into action."

Another patient speaks up, who worked for years as an elementary schoolteacher. "My doctor helped tremendously. He stuck by me through my initial anger about the diagnosis, then pointed out how many options for treatment there were. That gave me courage. "The doctor is really important," the other patients murmur in agreement. The Tunisian patient breaks through this chorus: "Yes, the doctor is very important, but your own heart is more important—it must want to fight for life, regardless of whether it succeeds or not."

Spirituality—Hope in Hopeless Times

Medicine is a natural science; it can and must follow its own tendencies. This means that the effects of medical procedures must be both verifiable and repeatable. Doctors who practice and research, such as myself, follow the principles of "evidence-based medicine," which seeks to determine the true value of operations and medication for patients by meticulously and systematically analyzing any studies that are currently available for the issue at hand. Within this body of literature, there are reports for nearly every medical topic and disease, which consider the role of spiritual factors in healing. By contrast, no such works address the most important and frequently used medical measure our disposal: the doctor's appointment. Still, it is obvious that especially in existential situations, transcendent experience as well as faith, no matter what its object, can play an important role. In other words, both can help recipients process bad news.

As doctors, we should have the courage to ask patients about this aspect of their lives. In the moment, after all, the goal is to identify the recipient's personal sources of strength and to mobilize those sources in the interests of coping with the bad news and its consequences. To my mind, because spirituality ascribes meaning, it does not conflict with modern, research-based medicine. On the contrary, it can even enrich a medical approach, helping the doctor become more aware of themselves and their patient's spirituality, a subject that is rarely touched upon in doctor–patient conversations. A sense of spirituality can also make patients more accessible and help to build trust. Obviously, a doctor should not come across as a missionary or foist their own beliefs on the patient. Rather, as I have emphasized repeatedly, doctors can listen, learn something about their patients' spirituality, and bring this information to bear on further treatment.

I remember Sister Hannah clearly, a nun from the Franciscan cloister in Sießen outside of Ulm. Her personality was larger than life; I accompanied her in her fight against cancer for 8 years. While we would discuss medical matters often enough, we spoke much more about God, and how complicated the world can be. We trusted each other, and each sincerely appreciated the other's company. She loved being a nun and found fulfillment in the church's work with youth and adolescents. Despite numerous chemotherapy sessions, her cancer returned time and again. "Sister Hannah," I asked her at some point, "don't you ever doubt your faith when the cancer returns repeatedly and refuses to let go?"

"Doubt? I speak with God, of course, and try to understand my destiny. It's an emotional, honest conversation—how could a conversation be honest without emotions? I may be sad, angry, or sarcastic at times, but I've never doubted my faith. My conversation with God has helped me to better see myself. It's the conversation itself that has given me strength and optimism."

I Won't Give Up, after All

My assistant calls and asks when I can come to see my patient, who is waiting for the results from today's operation. She is a well-known fashion journalist whom I have grown close to over the past 3 years of treatment. A high point came several months ago when—despite ongoing chemotherapy treatment—she organized an extravagant fashion show to benefit the "Ovarian Cancer Foundation." Just this morning, we had attempted an abdominal incision to relieve her stomach from a tumor that was pressing on it, in order to allow a bleeding inflammation in her esophagus heal. Unfortunately, up to that point every other attempt involving medication or less-invasive procedures had failed. During the operation, we had tried everything we could, but the cancer was too advanced—there were so many hard, cancerous tumors in the way that we were unable to access her stomach. In the end, we had to end the operation; there was nothing we could do to help her.

My assistant asks if I will speak with the patient; he doesn't know what to say or how she might react. We go up to her room and find her lying in bed. Her best friend sits next to her. Both seem depressed, they know that the operation wasn't successful, as the gastric tube hasn't been removed from the patient's nose. I take the patient's hand, which is warm. Somehow this gives me courage. I look her in the eyes and say: "We tried everything, but it didn't work." I pause and see that she is beginning to tear up. I clasp her hand more tightly and try to think of something positive I can tell her. I use the silence to think it over, hoping that something will occur. Nothing does.

"So what happens now?" she asks, breaking the silence.

"Please give me some time to think," I say. "Let's meet tomorrow at 8, if you like. Right now I'm not in a position to give you an honest answer. We need a little distance from the moment, and I need more time in order to sort out which options we should discuss together."

She nods, and I have the feeling that she is grateful to end the conversation there and take time to digest this sad news with her closest friend. The assistant walks out with me into the hall and thanks me. "You can see that there are some situations in life where you can't simply gloss things over, where it's important to speak the truth and allow space to grieve," I reply.

The next morning, we continue the conversation. *How will she be today?* I wonder, hoping that somehow she's managed to get a good night's sleep. I walk in, and she looks better than yesterday. I sit down at her side; my assistants stay standing. The patient looks around and then asks the young assistants to stand where she can see them. *I don't like it when someone is behind me, either,* I think to myself. "How are you today?" is my first question to her. Realizing this may not be the best way to begin, I immediately add: "You don't have to answer if you don't like."

She smiles but doesn't say a word. This morning she has opted for bright red lipstick. I briefly go over her current situation, and then together we retrace all the highs and lows of her long medical history: she's had three complex operations in the past 8 years and three rounds of chemotherapy of more than 20 units applications. She was first diagnosed with ovarian cancer in 2012 and underwent a complex surgery of more than 10 hours followed by chemotherapy over a half year. Then the cancer came back. If this form of cancer returns, it normally does so within 5 years. With her it has been different, however, atypical: after more than 7 years, a CT scan revealed metastases in the peritoneum. When ovarian cancer recurs, it is usually no longer treatable; now it has come back twice. I repeat that the cancer isn't curable, and that at the end of the day the most important goal for any form of medical treatment should be quality of life—something only she can judge. She nods.

"In your particular situation, I should mention a variety of options, but you don't have to choose one immediately. Just listen to them, and if you don't understand something, ask. Agreed?"

"Agreed," she replies.

I explain the various medical possibilities: I talk about hospice, about exclusively treating for symptoms such as pain, and about various methods that, even if they work, can only stave off tumor growth for a short time, and that at the cost of side effects such as hair loss and increasing physical weakness. She has just begun her most recent round of chemotherapy, so we can't actually say yet whether the treatment has worked or not, or if the cancer cells are resistant to this medication, too. Even with the stomach issues caused by the cancer's growth, overall she has responded well to the treatment; her hair hasn't even fallen out during the treatment.

"How do you see the situation? What are your wishes and plans? What do you think we should do now?" I ask her, seeing that she has already struggled greatly with this question for some time now. "Do you want to decide with me now, or should we meet later?"

I am expecting a long pause, but she answers immediately: "I'll keep going of course, I won't give up. I'd like to continue with the cancer treatment, I'm sure about that!"

As though someone just uttered a magic spell, the glum expressions on the assistants' faces vanish immediately. I accept her decision—it is an easy one to understand, even if there is a difficult path ahead and the chances of lasting success aren't good. But I am happy to support her—we'll support her with everything we are capable of.

"You must promise me one thing, however: Today you have to write out a living will and lay out the boundaries for how far we should actually go if you are in a life-threatening scenario and can't decide for yourself." She promises to work on out with her friend, and thanks me for the assignment.

Finishing and Documenting the Conversation

Once you have reached the end of the conversation, briefly summarizing the main points and naming next steps can give patients an added sense of orientation. When doing so, practical matters should be the central focus, details like the next appointment or the name of the colleague that will be in charge of further treatment.

If it feels as though a second follow-up conversation still makes sense, ask the person affected if they would also like to do so. If it becomes clear only after the fact that a second conversation is still needed, an appointment should be scheduled promptly.

As with surgical interventions, after which an "operational protocol," or detailed account of the essential operational procedures and potential complications must be filled out, doctors should also prepare a "conversational protocol." Such a protocol can help other team members and medical figures (such as a family doctor) get their bearings and serve as a basis for subsequent conversations with the patient. These protocols also help anticipate other potential conflicts in communication, for example, a patient's objection that they had not been notified or informed.

Conversations that involve bad news also represent a cognitive and emotional challenge to the person conveying the news. Regardless of how stressful their last conversation may have been, doctors must often continue to look after other medical duties without pause—be it an operation, an examination, or another doctor–patient conversation. This applies, moreover, to many situations in which bad news is communicated: I think again of police, whose work is rarely finished when they ring the doorbell.

Debriefing can be an effective way to reduce stress in doctors, or anyone conveying bad news for that matter. The term *debriefing* comes from "briefing," which is used to describe a meeting in which information or instructions are given before something important occurs. In our case, debriefing refers to a type of assessment, as well as a joint analysis of the conversations and/or event. This can happen with other colleagues, but also alone—in my mind a debriefing doesn't have to be a strict evaluation of what went wrong, or proper analysis. Sometimes a ritual such as washing one's hands or going for a short walk is enough. Something of this kind can have preventative effects, reducing stress and averting "burnout."

Such debriefings are, or course, no substitute for professional accompaniment and supervision. They can improve the psychic health of the person sharing the difficult news tremendously; however, by giving space to their thoughts and feelings and allowing the person to clear their mind of them before moving on to the next thing. Ideally, of course, this would take place in a structured environment decoupled from the immediate event, as in a coaching session or a Balint group (named for the psychiatrist and psychoanalyst Michael Balint). Another possibility is a working group of 8–12 doctors who meet under the direction of a psychotherapist or psychoanalyst in order to analyze and learn from "difficult patient situations" in their day-to-day experience.

While these are all actually secondary steps that are removed from the immediate situation, they may still help people recuperate their psychic health and ability to work. It is still important to conclude—and be able to move past—one-on-one conversations with a similar type of debriefing. I still remember what an air traffic controller once told me about this topic: If someone undergoes a difficult situation at work, for example, a "near accident," they are immediately released from all other duties and someone else takes over the rest of their shift. A systematic analysis is then carried out, with no fines or reprimands for employees.

Unfortunately, the field of medicine is leagues behind this type of thinking. If a doctor finds himself in a difficult situation, a complication in surgery, say, or a hard conversation with an unsatisfying conclusion, he generally still has to complete his shift. Not only is this strenuous, it can also be harmful to patients. If a doctor isn't able to truly process a stressful situation, the unresolved conflict can lead to inappropriate behavior during the next meeting with the patient.

"Mommy Is Very Sick"

Breaking the news that someone's parent or parents have died surely counts as one of the most important and most difficult challenges that exist, even more so when that someone is a young child. Yet, what holds true for adults also applies in these cases: Whatever one says, it must be true.

Children pick up on much of what is happening around them—often more than adults assume. For that reason alone, it makes sense to involve them, to listen to what they have to say, and to take their feelings and concerns seriously, even if one worries about not always giving the best answer. In any event, it is more about one's attitude than individual words. Honesty and having the courage to explain things are both important in gaining children's trust. For children, parents are their pillars of stability that allow them to mature into stable adults themselves. This means that children often live with the feeling that their parents are invincible. Yet, even parents are not immune to serious, even life-threatening illnesses. In Germany alone, an estimated three million children currently find themselves in such a situation. Every year, an additional 200,000 children in Germany learn that dad or mom is sick with cancer.

Uncertainty about the best way to break difficult news to children is as widespread among doctors as it is in families. One study showed that even when children were present at these conversations, they were hardly ever addressed, while scarcely one-half of children were informed separately of a parent's life-threatening illness, and younger children were seldom given an explanation about what was happening.

For their part, parents also often avoid this conversation with their kids—sometimes consciously, sometimes unconsciously. Symptoms from the disease or treatment may simply leave a patient feeling too weak to muster the strength for the difficult conversation; they are either too afraid themselves to speak about death or dying or are unsure of how to think about or describe their own medical situation. To my mind, grown-ups also have this right to restraint—at least for a little while. Parents also have a responsibility toward their children: to make sure they are not suddenly confronted with the parent's death unprepared, with no opportunity to say goodbye.

Children notice very quickly when something is wrong, that mom or dad is weaker, needs to rest more, and more often is not as active socially, or has to visit the hospital or doctor's office more and more frequently. Children need age-appropriate guidance from adults; this happens with open communication about the illness and encouraging children to ask questions. In lieu of questions being asked and answered out loud, children will often develop their own theories, believing, for example, that they are responsible for the disease. These theories then lead to ideas or images that scare them and have little basis in reality.

Children have their own way of dealing with information of this sort, and their reactions may differ greatly from those of grown-ups. Crying might be one response; anger, a wish to retreat, or self-expression in the form of painting, movement, or distraction are other responses. Even if these types of reactions are unfamiliar, parents and doctors alike should learn about and accept them, rather than feeding children catchphrases like "big boys don't cry."

To raise awareness within the medical profession for the particular care needed when discussing serious diagnoses with children, doctors should regard and address patients with children of their own first and foremost as parents. A number of different studies have shown, for example, that oncologists rarely initiate conversations with children. Perhaps these doctors feel conflicted because it is only the father or mother who is their patient, and not the other family members. At the same time, doctors should not feel as though it is their exclusive obligation to have conversations with each member of the family. Often, the necessary level of trust is lacking to make this a sensible idea in the first place. Doctors can, however, point to professional resources for assistance, and take advantage of those same resources themselves.

Children of Somatically Ill Parents (COSIP) has proved itself within a wide range of medical and social professions as an effective model for child-centered family counseling. It offers a theoretical groundwork as well as practical advice for planning and shaping consultations that bring together adult cancer patients, their children, and the extended family. Developed and tested simultaneously in Hamburg, Berlin, Heidelberg, Magdeburg, and Leipzig, the model usually consists of three to eight counseling sessions with conversations between parents, their children, and any siblings or extended family. The sessions focus on everyday life, and also examine the specific resources and needs that children have within the family. Taking a largely preventative approach, the conversations look to strengthen the patient's role as a parent.

Family goals during counseling might include more open communication about the parent's illness and supporting the parent's self-assurance and emotional availability. For children, goals might include greater cognitive orientation, legitimizing their own feelings and needs, and supporting a preliminary grieving process.

Unless they explicitly say otherwise—which should also be respected—children should be included in preparations to grieve and/or any rituals of grief that occur. Incorporating children in such rituals can give them a better handle on what's happening as well as a sense of security, which they will remember as a sort of mental milestone in their own grieving process. What we experience as children stays with us, later influencing how we react to bad news or twists of fate as adults.

This issue matters outside the hospital, too. I have been personally confronted with this very topic by my own children: it was a classic fall day bursting with red-browns and dark greens, it was just a few months before my mother passed away. We were driving along the Landwehr Canal listening to a mix of popular songs from the Arab world, when my daughter Sara, then aged 9 years, suddenly asked me to turn down the music—she had a question. "Will Grandma Aziza die soon?" she asked cautiously. Over the past several weeks, my mother's chronic heart failure and diabetes had led her back to the hospital more and more. "I don't know Sara, I hope not," I replied. "We have to pray for Grandma Aziza." She looked out the window for a few seconds, then turned back: "Dad, you can turn the music up again now!"

Examples from Outside Medicine

The Father and the Young Policeman

It's Thursday around 10 P.M. on a beautiful spring evening when the phone rings at police dispatch in Brandenburg: a car has crashed into a large tree on Birkenallee, and three people have been injured. Policeman Andreas Dalke drives to the site immediately; fortunately the streets are empty.

Minutes after the accident, three ambulances arrive at the scene. Andreas Dalke, the officer in charge, also shows up; he wants to get an idea of the accident for himself. The paramedics have already left by the time he gets there. Officer Mischke has been with the police for 26 years—at the secured site he meets Peter Zardo, a truck driver on his way to Prague. Peter has been on the road for over 7 hours, but his pale face shows no signs of weariness. He studied communications in Potsdam and speaks excellent German.

Peter describes how a red passenger car tried to pass him at a high speed. Focusing on the curve in the road, he only glimpsed the car at the last minute. "I saw a flash of light in the rearview mirror—when I looked into the side view mirror it had disappeared. Then I watched the tragedy unfold, just like in a movie. The car skidded, slid off the highway, and crashed into a tree on the right. It happened so quickly, for a moment I thought it couldn't be true, that I had fallen asleep and it was all a bad dream. It was unreal. The force of the crash split the car into two, I didn't hear anything. The front part of the car skidded over the wet highway toward the left, where it crashed into another tree."

He continued, "Meanwhile the rear part of the car continued sliding, flipped over twice, then crashed into a second tree. I almost drove off the road myself, but somehow I managed to stop the truck, then ran over to the scene. It was maybe only a hundred meters, but it felt like it took an eternity to get there.

"In the middle of the road lay a young man who wasn't moving. There was someone else in the rear part of the car, pinned in between the tree and the backseat—it was a young woman. She wasn't moving either. I called the fire department in a panic and tried to resuscitate the man. I pressed against his chest and kept watching his bloody face, hoping that he would wake up and wave me aside. I hoped somebody else would pass by, but no one else seemed to be out.

"About 20 meters away from the front section of the car, I heard a man lying in a cornfield, screaming. The ambulances arrived before I could figure out what to do. Sadly, though, the paramedics couldn't save anyone, everybody was hurt so badly that they all died. There was nothing else I could have done, right?!"

The man grows sadder and paler as he talks; now he wants to drive on, anywhere but here.

The police don't find any identification on the victims or in the remains of the destroyed passenger car. A license check reveals that the car was registered to an 18-year-old man from Hamburg. The policeman on site calls dispatch control and is transferred to the police station in Eppendorf. After describing the awful incident to his colleague on the other end of the line, the policeman requests that someone inform the nearest relatives of the deceased.

Thomas Maggler is on duty tonight, his fourth night patrol in the last 4 weeks. "One more night," he says to a new colleague who just passed his exams 4 weeks ago, "and then the day after tomorrow I can finally go see the doctor. These damned headaches keep getting worse." He has barely finished the sentence when they receive a call from central: "Car 274, please report!"

"Yes, 274 here."

"Please inform the parents of a deceased traffic accident victim, name Sven Lidzke, resides in Eppendorfer Straße."

The younger colleague recoils. "What? We have to tell the man's relatives that he died? Who are they?"

"The parents of the victim, Maria and Erwin Lidzke."

Both policemen take a deep breath, then finally turn right onto the busy street. After radioing in a patrol car and receiving some additional information, the two young colleagues make their way to the home of the victim's parents; by now it is 11:30 P.M. They have to ring the bell five times before a window opens on the second floor and a bare-chested man looks out: "What is it now?" he says, looking down as though he's gone through this before.

"Open up please, we have to speak with you," says the older policeman. A few seconds later, the electric door buzzes. The policemen enter and meet the father in the hall.

"We have some bad news for you, but first we have to ask you a few questions. Can we come upstairs with you?"

"No!" the father stammers loudly, "I want to know what's going on right now!"

"Do you want to call your wife?" the policeman continues.

"Let her sleep, she has Parkinson's, and she's not doing well right now. She's on heavy medications and hasn't been able to get any rest. Right now she's sleeping more soundly than she has for months."

Slowly and carefully, the older policeman attempts to explain what happened. "There was a serious accident," he begins. The younger policeman looks down at the ground in embarrassment. "Do you know where your son is or what his plans were?"

The father replies that his son left around 6 P.M. to go to a rock concert in Berlin with his girlfriend and a local friend. "My son loves rock concerts," the father says to the younger policeman, who looks up for a minute. "My son also loves his Volkswagen Golf. He doesn't let anybody else drive his precious car, not even me, though I paid for the whole thing."

The son only left the house that afternoon, so the father can give a precise description of his clothing; everything checks out. The older policeman takes a deep breath, then says: "It was a really bad accident. I'm sorry, but I have to inform you that your son is dead."

The father collapses, breaking out in tears. "I knew it, the first time you rang, I knew it, it was that damned souped-up car, I just knew it!" He screams, banging against the elevator door, first with his fists, then with his head. He cuts his head and begins to bleed from his forehead, continuing to scream. The younger policeman calls an ambulance and then dials the number for the crisis intervention team and emergency welfare. He looked up the numbers ahead of time and has them at the ready. The phone rings for a long time, but no one answers; he tries various numbers but is too shaky to enter the digits correctly. Wrong number, he keeps hearing. The father is panting and grows paler, then faints. Both policemen try to catch the man as he falls to the ground but don't make it in time, and he hits his head on the stairwell floor. The younger policeman checks the father's breathing.

"He's breathing, thank God. When will the ambulance finally get here?"

In the Train

I am on the train from Berlin to Rostock, watching it rain outside the window and thinking of Thomas—a close friend who held a post a while back as a professor at a prestigious university hospital. Always ready with a smile, today he's deeply involved in work in Africa, where he sends me regular updates about his wonderful experiences in Kenya and Morocco. Several years ago, he was forced to resign from his post, after he was accused of making errors in treating patients. He had to endure, then comment on, countless reports in the press. "The looks of the purported witnesses are more difficult than the words my colleagues have left unspoken," I remember him telling me.

We meet at a cancer conference in Chicago, Illinois, and I ask him about that time. "Yes, that was a very difficult period," he replies smiling, looking at me as though he were proud of not having lost his joy in life.

"What helped you to manage when you were told that you couldn't stay on as the hospital head?" I ask.

"We finally managed to come to an agreement, but it was really difficult for me. I knew that the academic career I loved so much was over forever, after 40 years of studying how to improve treatment results in patients. My wife helped tremendously. She stayed by my side and encouraged me not to give up. Soon enough, I started hoping that I might be able do something meaningful again, even without my position as a head doctor. Something that would help people. I know now that was entirely possible, but at the time I had serious doubts about whether I would succeed. I didn't know anything else other than science. I think I might even be doing better today than before, but it has taken years."

Work, career, and professional status often dominate our lives. This means the workplace is a common setting in which recipients receive news with existential implications. This could, of course, be a good thing—additional employees, for example, or more free time for one's private life. It could just as easily be bad news, however, or news that is perceived negatively and may trigger anger or frustration. A promotion one had counted on being given to someone else, for example, a vacation that isn't granted, or even a dismissal. I have personally experienced how strongly people react when, for example, they hear that their contract hasn't been extended, perhaps because their personality isn't a good match for the team or because their goals and values don't match hospital leadership. Early in my career, I also felt hurt when colleagues decided to leave work before their contract was over, because they wanted to change practices or move to another hospital. It is essential to explain a decision to release somebody in a transparent way, and to make it clear that it isn't about a complete rejection of the person but is happening for multiple reasons. This is a way of showing respect for the person even if their professional skills are not adequate for the job. The way in which a company or a team fires employees, moreover, sends a strong signal to remaining colleagues.

Rumors often circulate quickly among remaining staff before, but at the latest shortly after an employees' termination becomes known. This can traumatize an entire team, or at least unsettle it. That's why it is advisable to inform the entire staff—not just leadership—once the bad news has been shared with the person. The employee in question should, as a matter of course, always be the first to find out about their termination. If possible, avoid firing somebody without advance warning, where employees aren't given the chance to say goodbye to each other. Not being able to say goodbye is often talked about as leaving lasting injury and causing psychological damage. Employees who don't want a farewell party should at least receive a small personal gesture, a card wishing them well, for example. As with breaking bad medical news, one hears about how it helps people to hear the truth immediately and directly, face to face, instead of beating about the bush.

Sometimes the person doing the firing may agonize for a long time over a "poorly" delivered dismissal, especially if this came about at one's own discretion, as a part of business restructuring, for example. As with doctor–patient conversations, personal business coaches first advise delivering the message clearly and unmistakably. Then pause and allow room for silence. As I've discussed for doctors, once you've delivered the bad news, try and resist the urge to fill every lull in the conversation with other unnecessary remarks, simply in order to avoid uncomfortable silences. Your employee has just found themselves in an emotionally difficult moment and needs time to gather their thoughts in silence. Allow the employee to react, accept, and bear with feelings like disappointment or anger. In such situations, it may also make sense to schedule a follow-up meeting instead of squeezing every last formality and detail into a single conversation and risk overwhelming the recipient. Be empathetic and try to imagine the person's situation. In this context, it can help to get a sense of your counterpart's social environment and emotional state ahead of time. Another tip: If at all possible, a conversation that involves dismissing somebody shouldn't happen on Friday afternoon. The person may need professional or personal assistance or want to contact a lawyer, which can absolutely help with processing a termination.

In another parallel to doctor–patient conversations and what we have seen with police, one recent study from business consultants Kienbaum estimated that around 70% of business leadership in Germany are not prepared to lead these kinds of conversations with employees. In all three fields, continued professional training on breaking bad news is neither comprehensive nor required.

Nontransparent dismissals, or conversations that are perceived as unfair by the employee, can also lead to work arbitration trials and have unnecessary negative consequences for customers and one's own employees. Acting respectfully through the end of employment can also pay off in the future, as it is entirely possible the person will either be rehired or will show up again in a different professional setting. Just as a doctor doesn't simply leave a patient to their fate after delivering a diagnosis, one could formulate a general rule for the business world: don't lead only within your organization, but also outside of it. Throughout my own career, I have seen numerous cases of colleagues or professional coworkers who return to the team with greater motivation than before and are welcomed back with open arms. Try and open yourself—and your employees—to a similar possibility and perspective.

3

On the Search for Good News

CONTENTS

I'm boarding the plane to Cologne, where in several hours I'm scheduled to give a talk to a group of young doctors. The flight is already delayed, and we're still waiting for several passengers. The inevitable feeling of rush and stress fills the room as the passengers suddenly begin to push toward the gate—as though they might arrive sooner if they are the first on the plane. The last passenger to board, however, appears completely relaxed as he takes his seat, wearing a pair of comfortable jeans and a pair of headphones around his neck. *Here's a man who knows how to deal with stress*, I think to myself, *and who doesn't let anxiety rub off on him. It's sympathetic. And healthy.* This thought has barely occurred when I recognize him: it's Eckart von Hirschhausen, probably Germany's best-known doctor, as well as a cabaret artist, moderator, and bestselling author. I'm delighted to be sitting next to him. We know people in common and have a fair amount to discuss as colleagues, discussing humor in medicine and exchanging experiences and stories. Von Hirschhausen has made it his job to talk about communication, which of course I find fascinating, and he also finds something to take from my anecdotes.

It is an intensive, stimulating conversation—the well-loved comedian is distracted only briefly by the quick, fluid motions of the flight attendant issuing safety instructions. Von Hirschhausen does a professional imitation—a regular occurrence from the looks of it—following her gestures nearly simultaneously. The attendant smiles but keeps her composure, finishing the announcement with another quick grin. This much we can agree on: "Medicine can smile and laugh without losing its gravity or professionalism." He talks to me about his organization, "Humor Helps Healing" (*Humor Hilft Heilen*), which as a part of its program sends clowns into hospitals to act out funny stories with cancer patients nearing the end of their illness. He tells me about a friend of his with a very advanced case of intestinal cancer. His friend's doctor reported a 95% mortality rate in similar cases; the friend allowed the oncologist to finish speaking, then replied: "Doctor, you've spoken at great length about the 95% chance of bad results, now I'd like to hear something about the other 5%."

Changing Perspective

I'm watching the 8 o'clock news as do nine million others every day, seeing one horror story play out after the other. A tragic highway accident involving a family with three young children between Nuremberg and Regensburg, a bomb attack in Libya, a reactor failure in Japan. Even the sports and the weather are negative; Germany lost to the Czech Republic, and it's supposed to rain all day. Speaking in his lovable Dutch accent, the popular television host Rudi Carrell observes ironically, but accurately, how "News hosts always begin by saying 'Good Evening,' then take 15 minutes explaining why it isn't a good evening at all."

Is there really no good news at all that is worth reporting on? *We need a change of perspective, in medicine and society,* I think to myself. From a very early age it seems, we are socialized to watch for bad news, with anything that is bad or turns out badly being called to our attention. We are trained to search for errors in seemingly lighthearted images: what's wrong here, where are the mistakes hidden? Why are we trained to look for the mistakes in what we see?

Now that we have spent some time exploring the question of how to communicate bad news, we should turn to good news. Every day, countless diagnostic tests are performed: ultrasounds, computed tomography (CT) scans, magnetic resonance imaging (MRI) scans, and so on. Blood values are also tested: potassium, sodium, creatinine, urea, liver enzymes, erythrocytes, leukocytes, platelets, and much more. One often observes doctors concentrating on abnormal results in their visits; any "good news" is simply not expressed. One often hears statements such as "your potassium levels are low, we have to give you an infusion." By contrast, one rarely hears, "the blood values we tested for yesterday which measure the functioning of the kidneys, liver, and bone marrow all came out great." This happens despite the fact that ill patients are desperately looking for good news, like someone dying of thirst searching for water in the desert.

Shouldn't we all be prepared for bad news, though? Sooner or later, everyone will presumably confront it at least once in their lives, if not more. While we can't prevent bad news, we can at least prepare, and in doing so it helps a great deal if one has positive stories about easy conversations to turn to. To do so, however, we have to approach sharing good news with the same amount of intention as we do when we are breaking bad news. Good news can give us strength and connect us to life and our love of living.

Bad news travels fast and more easily than good news does—it's quantifiable. But what is the cause for this? In one large-scale study in the United States, a quarter of participants named stress as the reason for their current state of ill-ease. The most common causes of this stress were bad news from the Internet, television, radio, and newspapers. Bad news also has the power to make people sick. Another study surveyed 4500 people about their reactions to the terror attacks at the Boston Marathon. Those who spent more than 6 hours watching the news about the terrorist act showed the most acute symptoms of stress—even more than people who were present at the scene of the bombing. Maybe newscasters, similar to a doctor announcing a cancer diagnosis, should first warn their audience before delivering bad news, then pause briefly to prepare them. This could weaken, although probably not eliminate, any negative psychological effects.

Simply pointing a finger at the media, however, seems overly simplistic and wrongheaded. Concentrating on bad news while taking little account of good news is not a new phenomenon. Bad news seems to get attention and be passed on more easily. "It's what the people want," news channels say. If that is the case, then why? "All prejudices come from the intestines," Nietzsche writes. Is it that negative news confirms and serves biases and fears we acquired in early childhood more than good news does? Is it easier to deal with bad news than it is to feel empathy and joy over good news? Does bad news about others help us feel better about our own lives? It may also be a question of time: it takes longer and requires greater attention and free time for sympathy and hope to develop than for fear, disgust, or anger to develop. Good news tends to be "slow" news, by which I mean its effects take longer to unfold but also usually last longer than whatever bad news there is currently. I've never heard of someone being shocked by good news. Is it that our society has simply forgotten the experience of showing surprise at good news?

We should try to free ourselves from unnecessarily obsessing over negative news. By this I don't mean forced optimism, but rather a sense for recognizing and distinguishing good news among the difficult outcomes and prospects that life sends in our direction.

The Good Evening News

For a long time now, I've brought each day in the hospital to a close by visiting one of my patients and bringing them some good news. I'm constantly surprised at how easy it is to find something to say. I don't have to invent good news, nor would I—the key word here is "truthfulness." Once one begins to think about it, it seems to come just as naturally as difficult news. It is an entirely personal effort I make not to simply give in to bad news, but also to value good news in appropriate measure.

Good news is empowering; it generates positive feelings and strengthens the patient's beleaguered self-consciousness. What's more, it increases the level of satisfaction I feel with my work as a doctor; I simply need to stay aware of it. I am determined to celebrate and enjoy good news to the full with my patients. It also strengthens my resilience as a doctor: it has become easier to withstand the bad or difficult situations that form a part of everyday life at the hospital. My sleep has improved. Looking back on my day, it is much easier to see than it is during the daily grind that there are many more pieces of good news doctors learn about every day—and could pass on to their patients—than pieces of bad news they are forced to communicate.

What I've written about pauses and silence when sharing bad news also applies for happier pieces of information. Good news also takes time and space to sink in; one needs to come to terms with and process positive messages. Recently, I said to one patient, "That was a highly complex and invasive 6-hour operation, I'm so glad that you handled it as well as you did." I paused briefly for about 5 seconds. She began to cry and hugged me without saying a word. The good news had really reached her; it hadn't gotten lost.

Good news can be particularly powerful when it is delivered in a group setting. The word "relatives" immediately conjures thoughts of dying, death, and grief. Yet, relatives can also be there with us when we expect, or at least hope for good news.

Breaking Good News!

Anna, a close friend of mine, is also a doctor. She originally wanted to study art history and has loved painting for as long as she can remember. Her favorite subject is birds. She became a doctor for her parents, who are doctors themselves, each with their own practices. Her father was a heart specialist; her mother was a well-loved dermatologist. Anna spent every free minute she had painting, although working as an emergency medic with more than seven night shifts each month didn't leave many opportunities. At one point, she learned about a gallery in Berlin's Schöneberg that was planning an exhibition of new female artists. For a long time, she debated whether to apply or not; on the one hand, she wanted finally to receive some affirmation for her artistic talent, but she was also afraid of being disappointed if she were turned down. She ended up submitting three paintings to the gallery and was told it would take about 7 days for the works to be judged. That entire week Anna threw herself into work in an effort to distract herself, but to no avail. Finally, she heard back: "We're happy to inform you that your paintings have been selected by an independent jury to be included in our next exhibition." She was so happy that she cried, like she never had before. She immediately wanted to celebrate the good news with her sister and parents but couldn't reach anyone when she tried calling—not even her best friend. What had been feelings of pure bliss soon became tinged with sadness and loneliness.

While Anna still felt happy, she was sad about not being able to share the news with the people who mattered the most to her. Based on this experience, she resolved to always try and be present for, and take genuine pleasure in the happiest moments in the lives of the people who mattered to her. For her, it became very clear that these were just as important to share as moments of pain, or difficult turns of fate.

Good news can also act as a buffer to help absorb pain or fear and help us classify or dampen the effects of bad news. Sooner or later, the moment will come to us all—we can't determine the point in time, but we can prepare for it and draw from the good experiences in our lives. Good news can give us strength and connect us to life and our love of living. Sharing good experiences or news gives us the necessary strength to resist the unforeseen or fateful; they give us the strength to face whatever bad news life brings.

The Chess Flower

It's Tuesday, and time for my weekly visit to the wards as head doctor. We have just finished discussing at our tumor conference the CT scan of a 53-year-old patient who was transported by ambulance to the hospital yesterday. Her left leg had suddenly swollen up, she had difficulty breathing, and she had exhaustion. Several days before, she had received the second cycle of chemotherapy. She had dealt with the increasing weakness from the first cycle well; there had been no nausea or vomiting, although her long dark hair had fallen out. The current diagnosis was pulmonary embolism due to deep vein thrombosis and multiple lung metastases due to leiomyosarcoma. Leiomyosarcoma is a rare and aggressive form of uterine cancer. Because the cancer had already spread to the patient's lungs, she was being treated with chemotherapy instead of receiving an operation.

And now a blood clot in the lungs. A colleague stops me as I am about to enter the patient's room: "She doesn't know yet, Doctor." I look at her thankfully and then open the door and walk over to her bed, trailed by two other doctors, the ward nurse, and a nutritionist. She's alone in the room. I offer her my hand and ask: "How's it going?"

The patient seems happy to have us there. "I'm doing well today," she replies in a clear voice. I had spoken with her briefly a couple days before, and she hadn't been doing nearly as well.

"How's your breathing?" I continue.

"Also much better."

"And your leg?"

"The swelling is going down; the blood thinners seem to be doing their job, Doctor."

I try to explain to her that the blood clot in her lungs represents a critical situation, and that she should use physical therapy to improve her lung function and avoid inflammation. "I've already walked two flights of stairs today and have been using the breathalyzer a lot." She points to the TriFlo, a small device that one breathes into to try and move three small balls.

"When a blood clot appears in cases of cancer, it's often a sign that the cancer has continued to grow despite the chemotherapy," I say, then pause. She looks up at me; no one speaks. After about 5 seconds, she says, "Well then, just operate and take out the cancer once and for all."

Without commenting on this appeal for the moment, I talk instead about the conclusions from our tumor conference, in which different representatives from various disciplines such as pathology, radiotherapy, and gynecology discuss a patient's treatment options in detail. I take a deep breath and force myself to speak slowly: "The exam we performed after your blood clot and respiratory problems also showed lung metastases. Unfortunately, the results aren't good."

Pause.

"That's what I thought, Doctor, so an operation doesn't make any sense, right?"

"That's right, an operation doesn't make sense, because the cancer colonies in the lungs are now our main focus," I reply.

"What can we do?" She asks.

"It's a very difficult situation. In principle we could switch to another form of cancer treatment, but there isn't a cure."

She looks out the window for a moment. "What will the treatment do then?" she asks.

"At best, alleviate your symptoms for a while, and slow the tumor's growth."

"And how long is 'a while'?" she persists.

"Every case is different. For some, several weeks; for others it can be months."

"And what about the side effects?"

"Most respond well to the treatment, although there is no effect without a side effect," I reply. "Physical weakness, nausea, and anemia are the most common."

"And what can I do on my own against these side effects?"

"As a first step, be prepared and let your doctor know about any if they appear," I reply. "Get a lot of fresh air and regular physical activity, eat healthy, work against the physical weakness, and spend time with the people whom you love and will support you. That's my advice."

"And what are the alternatives to such a difficult form of treatment?" she asks.

"It is fully within your rights not to pursue chemotherapy, choosing not to spend your remaining time coping with the side effects from the treatment."

She looks at me again. "Doctor, thanks for your explanations, I'm a bit tired now."

I offer to continue the conversation tomorrow, once she's had a chance to discuss what she has just learned with her family. She looks off to the side for a moment, then turns back quickly and says: "No, I had decided to continue with cancer treatment even before this conversation. What you just explained to me strengthened my conviction, for that I'm grateful to you." I'm somewhat surprised but try not to let it show.

"What's the worse news you've received in your life?" I want to know. Somehow, she seems unsurprised by the question; she ponders for a moment, then answers, "I couldn't say, it hasn't been all that bad up to now."

"Then what about the best news you've ever received?" She seems to take this question in stride as well. "I couldn't tell you that, either," she replies.

My colleagues, the nurse, and the nutritionist are all somewhat unnerved by the patient's inability to think of an answer. A strange feeling settles in the sterile hospital air, as though important medical findings had been kept secret during the visit. I finish by asking the patient to think about my last two questions and tell her that I will come to check on her next week during my visit.

I hurry down the four flights of stairs on my way to the outpatient clinic on the ground floor, where two patients are waiting for me. The steps are smooth; it looks as though they've just been washed. I have to take care not to slip, but I am still distracted by the patient's two unanswered questions. I repeat each to myself: "What was the worst news you've ever received in your life? What was the best news?" I'm two floors away; my footsteps echo in the hallway. The questions change in my mind, and I begin to ask myself: "What was the worst news I've received in my life? What was the best?" I slow down—the questions slow me down. I think about it but find that I don't want to answer right away, I want to take my time. Maybe I don't want to answer them in the first place. I reach the outpatient clinic—the younger patient is accompanied by her mother, while the older, 73-year-old patient is there with her husband. I open the door and invite the older patient into the conference room first.

We've known each other for a long time now and greet each other warmly. She's doing better—as we sit down I ask her somewhat abruptly, "What was the best news you've received in your life up to now?"

"The birth of my daughter!" She replies immediately.

"And yours?" I say, turning to her husband, who is maybe 2 or 3 years older than his wife. His face bears all the traces of a long life; he's also had two heart attacks and been operated on for colon cancer.

"The best news—it must have been late summer 1942, when a Russian soldier screamed "*blin Hitler*" at me, which I guess meant "damn Hitler," then emptied his rifle above me into the attic of an old house. He let me live."

"And what was the worst news?" I ask him.

"My wife being diagnosed with ovarian cancer," he replies without hesitating. I look to his wife who merely smiles, as though she knew ahead of time what the answer would be.

I excuse myself, thanking each for their forthright answers. I am beginning to see more and more that it is less about the news itself than it is about the events. I ask for news, and they answer with a description of a moving moment, or intense experiences. Perhaps instead of "breaking bad news," we should call it "being present at difficult life situations?"

Focusing on the news alone may very well end up preventing us from fully appreciating the event or its impact on the recipient's life. By this I do not mean delving into all of the potential difficulties and problems, which would only increase the person's feeling of dread. Rather, it is much more about recognizing that while the current conversation is a very important one, it will ultimately take its place as one in a series of important conversations. Paying attention to this can help to reduce stress on the current conversation, as not everything must be solved all at once. Try not to set too much weight on the discussion but spread it over multiple appointments and multiple actors. Give the person with whom you have to share the bad news time to take a break from carrying the weight—do the same for yourself. Concentrate on the conversation, but also on how you can help lift the recipient's burden instead of just bearing it—how to help the recipient take active steps.

It's the young patient's turn now. Her mother enters the room first, as though looking to make sure it is safe for her daughter. We have some radiological test results to discuss—several days ago she visited her gynecologist for pain she had felt for a while, and her cervix had looked highly suspicious. A tissue sample confirmed the fears: it was cervical cancer. We had conducted subsequent tests to clarify whether the cancer had already spread, and whether an operation, radiation, or chemotherapy will be necessary. The tumor measures 5 cm. The patient works as a kindergarten teacher and badly wants children for herself. I ask her about the best news she's received in her life as well, trying to give her plenty of time to think about it. She thinks for a moment but can't answer the question, nothing occurs at her young age. "And the worst news?" I ask. "This diagnosis," she says quietly.

I read through the test results, looking for the assessment paragraph. Everyone is tense—the mother, the patient, even I feel it. Line by line, the tension diminishes. There are no signs of metastases. I look to the patient, whose eyes have filled with tears. She doesn't say a word, waiting for my "translation."

"All your organs and lymph nodes are without any pathological results," I tell her. She breaks out in tears of joy.

"*That's* the best news I've had in my whole life!" Everyone relishes this beautiful moment and wants to hold onto it.

"Professor, can I tell you about the best news I've ever had?" the patient's mother asks, still with tears in her eyes. I nod. "It was when my son was born. He had just come into the world but didn't make a sound. I remember there was this frightening silence in the room. Everyone was waiting for him to scream, for my baby to draw his first breath, but none came. The silence grew heavier and heavier, everyone was really worried. We all looked at him, terrified—and what did he do? He peed all over the midwife's arm and started screaming. That was my best news!"

That evening on my way home, I wonder whether we sometimes have to live through bad news or difficult moments before our sense and understanding of what is good and positive is sharpened. How significant does good news have to be for us to take notice? Doesn't every piece of news deserve acknowledgment?

It's Tuesday again—today I'm meeting the leiomyosarcoma patient, whom I asked to think about my questions. She's in Room 14, right in the middle of the ward. I briefly consider beginning my rounds in Room 14, but the thought has barely crossed my mind when I decide against it: *No, keep to the usual routine despite your curiosity,* I think, *if only out of respect for the other patients. How would you explain starting in the middle to your coworkers, anyway?* Although I've begun any number of visits in particular rooms, the patients in those cases had medical issues like sudden respiratory problems or intense pain; in this case, my curiosity would be the only reason for changing my ritual.

Rituals make a lot of sense in everyday life at a hospital, although they should not all simply be adopted or left unchanged. Quite the opposite is true—many medical rituals are misinformed. This time, however, I stick with my typical beginning point in Room 1. After about 30 minutes, we've reached Room 14. The patient seems to have been expecting us. I ask her how she is. Her breathing is noticeably better, and the swelling in her leg has decreased. "How are her other blood values?" I ask the assistant.

"They're very good. The anemia has also subsided."

"That means we can plan the next cancer treatment, right?" I ask both the patient and my coworker. They answer at the same time, almost as if they had practiced: "Yes."

"Good. In that case, I recommend that we begin treatment tomorrow or the day after. The doctor can discuss all the details with you after our visit," I add.

"Doctor, you had given me another assignment," the patient tells me.

"That's right, although it was less an assignment than a favor," I reply. "Did you think of anything?"

She smiles and asks me to look behind the window curtain. "You'll find my answer at the window." I draw back the curtain and see, next to vases filled with carnations and tulips, a plant still wrapped in paper. The plant has a bell-shaped purple flower with a striking chessboard pattern on its pedals; I also see a card hanging from it. "Please take this plant and read the few lines I wrote." I thank her, and we step out of the room.

Outside, I read the card. "Thank you so much for your direct questions. I've asked myself them many times before but without fully realizing, it seems. This plant, the chess flower is my gift to you. I picked it first because it is threatened with extinction, so it speaks to the vulnerability of nature and life. But it also reminds me of the black and white pattern on a chessboard, which goes along well with my answer: There can't be a black and white answer to your questions—at most it's about the contrast."

Finding the Good in the Bad—A Question of Timing

As one study showed impressively, peoples' initial emotional reaction to news and their later course of action depend importantly on what they hear first. The last thing that is communicated stays in the memory longer than what was first communicated. Angela Legg and Kate Sweeny from the University of California in Riverside conducted one interesting experiment: In the study, one-half of participants were asked to give the other members of the group immediate feedback on a test in which both positive and negative results were presented to each subject. Although 78% of recipients preferred to hear the bad news before the good news, 54% of people stated they would prefer to share good news before bad news. These results show yet again that recipients would rather find out any bad news first in order to face it. For their part, those breaking the news tend to share any good news first in order to try and prepare their counterparts—and maybe themselves—for what is to come.

In a further experiment, subjects were asked to place themselves in the position of their counterpart. Following this change in perspective, those breaking the bad news found they did want to hear the bad news first. In a final experiment, the researchers examined how the order of the news affected recipients' behavior (self-criticism, willingness to learn from mistakes). They concluded that overall, recipients felt better when they heard the good news last. If, however, the important part was to draw personal lessons from the bad news, it was better to communicate the bad news *after* the good.

Today I met with the husband of a patient. He is a rabbi, a wonderful human being: wise and caring toward his wife, well read, a world traveler—and he speaks fluent Arabic. By now he has over 50 years of experience in helping and comforting people and providing them with answers to the difficult and beautiful moments of life. I asked him if he had ever had to share bad news with someone, and how that had been. He reflected for a moment, then replied that he wasn't usually the first person to share the bad news, but rather came in later to lend the person strength and assistance. He did remember one occasion: "The mother of a young man who was at his Bar-Mitzvah—the celebration of religious maturity in Judaism—once asked me to tell the son that just a few hours ago, his father had passed away unexpectedly."

"How did you go about telling this to the young man?"

"He was enjoying himself so much that I let him celebrate. He thought that his father had just gone home early because he had been ill with the flu for the past several days. His father wasn't in the habit of saying goodbye to anybody, not even his family. Later that evening, I went up to the son and told him that after this wonderful celebration, I now had some very sad news to tell him. His mother grew silent and took his hand. They didn't say another word for the rest of the evening and stayed close together. It was only the next day that they had to cry."

"And what helped the young man?" I asked.

"Later I met him and he told me that he was grateful for receiving the news of his father's death after his Bar-Mitzvah." Throughout the celebration, he imagined his father had also enjoyed himself, just like everybody else. "It was our party," he said.

Back at Office Hours

Professor Steinführer is back for a visit to my office hours. She is doing much better—she's responded extremely well to radiation, with no signs of side effects; no nausea, vomiting, or memory lapses. Still, she seems worn down. She had a CT scan taken yesterday, and today we're supposed to discuss the results. Her breathing has improved, which we hope is a sign that the lung metastases have stopped growing. Her brain metastases, on the other hand, did continue to grow during treatment—the breast cancer seems to have become resistant. We smile somewhat helplessly at each other, and then look at the radiologists' report together. There is a lot of text, and I search out the keywords: the thorax or chest, and pulmonary filiae, or lung metastases. The lung metastases haven't grown. They've even grown smaller, they are in remission!

We celebrate the good news for a little while as though we had been expecting it, then agree to continue the current antihormonal treatment and reevaluate the situation in 2 months, at which point we will also conduct another CT scan of her brain and lungs. We embrace, then search out the date for our next meeting.

4

Moscow

CONTENTS

I am in Moscow, an extraordinary city. What fantastic culture I've been missing out on. Following my presentation on the latest developments in cancer medicine and communication at the state hospital, a young doctor approaches me and asks in excellent German: "Doctor, may I ask you how one learns to speak with patients and share bad news with them?"

"Collect your patients' life stories—learn how to observe patients and ask them about what they find helpful in conversations, and what scares or weakens them. Ask about what happened after you had your conversation—that afternoon, the following day, the following month, and years later—what they remember, which colors, the feeling in the room. Compare this information with your own experiences and memories. Accompany your colleagues when they have to share difficult news, as well as good news. Learn more about grief and joy in patients, and search out your own answers."

That is the secret of the art of breaking bad news.

In Place of an Author's Biography: My Saddest, and Most Beautiful News

What about the exceptional moments of news in my own life? My mind seems to resist the search for concrete answers; thoughts flit quickly about before striking a familiar path marked by several keywords: mother, death, and admission to medical school.

Receiving news of the death of my mother was without doubt one of the most painful moments in my life. I don't really have to remember it at all—it's right there, burned into my mind. My father-in-law and I were on the way to a presentation at Berlin's Charité hospital. It was a quarter before nine and we were coming from Kreuzberg, where we had picked up my wife Adak. I remember that the spring gave the morning an odd color; we were listening to news from Berlin and around the world on the radio, although none of it seemed to be all that important. It grew darker and darker as we entered the tunnel that runs beneath Berlin's main train station; the radio signal faded gradually and then was lost. Suddenly, the cell phone rang. I glanced down at the screen and was surprised to see the name of my brother-in-law, Nabil, appear.

"He never calls this early," I said to my father-in-law. I turned down the radio until the voice of the newscaster faded off. I couldn't believe what he was saying to me. I didn't want to believe what he was telling me as softly as he was able. *It can't be true*, I cried out mournfully, repeating the words again and again. The car continued moving, but all I could do was watch out the window. I couldn't see anything; my lips were trembling. Adak looked at me as though she knew what had happened. I found myself wishing that the time before my brother-in-law had called would stand still, and for a moment it felt as though it might actually be possible. It was as though I were in a free fall. "What should I do?" I asked Adak candidly as we came out of the underpass. "You need to cancel the presentation and call your sister," she answered.

We pulled over, and I called my siblings: first my brother, then my sister. My sister wasn't able to speak either—my brother-in-law tried to get her on the phone but we couldn't manage. I had never heard her cry that way before. My oldest brother was also mute with grief. Without speaking, we were united in our grief. When I think about that phone call from my brother-in-law, the entire story comes up at once, not just individual fragments.

And the best news I've ever received? I don't have to think for long: it was a letter from the Freie Universität in Berlin. In school I held fast to my dreams of studying medicine, despite being repeatedly belittled by a number of teachers who said I wasn't good enough. Just like my mother, who was illiterate but spoke five languages and worked with great pride as a hospital ward assistant in Wedding, I was also in love with medicine. This might easily be because I spent nearly 6 months as a small boy in the hospital after a traffic accident, and was amazed at how the doctors healed me and the other children. It was a very scary period for me, especially when my cast needed to be changed. I screamed as loudly as I was able every time the doctor stood before me and my cast with a saw, and one of the nurses held me down. At the time, I remember thinking that the medical staff didn't have any doubts, a feeling of security that helped me greatly.

I continue to love medicine today. I still clearly remember one moment from my last year in high school. The biology teacher asked each student what he or she wanted to do after the final exams. My friend Güray wanted to be an engineer; Petra, the best in the class, wanted to be a pharmacist. Then it was my turn. "I want to study medicine" I said—I couldn't bring myself to admit that I wanted to be a doctor.

"Medicine?" The teacher asked with a dismissive smirk.

"Yes, medicine." I replied.

"My dear Jalid, I'm sorry to say it won't happen, not with a 3 in biology. It would be better to seek out another career." I didn't reply—what more could I have said?

I finished my exams with an average of 2.3 on a scale of 1.0 to 6.0—generally a good result. My entire family and I were very proud of the results; I had far and away the best grades among my group of friends. I was also a far cry, however, from the cutoff to be accepted to enter the medical university program, which at the time was an average of 1.3. I had heard about some students who registered for different courses of study like chemistry or physics, and then later switched over to medicine as "lateral entrants." To do that, however, it required a good deal of luck and patience to get permission to attend seminars and take exams independently. I was accepted into a law course but opted instead to pursue training as a nurse at the Rudolf Virchow Hospital, hoping to learn more about medicine. I still remember my first shifts as a nursing student at the "chronic wing," or what today we call the *geriatric ward*. Getting up early didn't come easily, but once we began to bathe patients at 6 A.M., I didn't mind it. What was difficult to overcome, however, was the smell of urine; it felt like the sharp scent stuck to me throughout the day and even followed me home. I complained to my mother, who listened patiently: "Mom I don't think I can make it through the training, the smell of the urine is so bad." My brother came into the room, carrying a large dark package with him. He was just about to open his first under- and oversized shoe store in Steglitz. "Good afternoon, my son," my mother said to him. "What's in the package?"

"Bottles of perfume, a lot of expensive perfume," he replied, setting the cardboard box down on the heavy marble table. Mom opened it and removed a bottle, and then a number of small samples. "Alain Delon," the label read. My mother looked at me and placed two samples in my hand. "Dab a couple of drops under your nostrils in the morning and see how it goes." I looked back at her skeptically but took the samples and waited to try the following day. It worked! These days I don't need perfume to work, but one thing has stayed with me: whenever I pass someone on the street wearing the same perfume, I'm reminded of the valuable time I spent at the geriatric station.

Some weeks later, I was invited for a selection interview at the Freie Universität. A miniscule number of places were assigned directly by the university by lottery, while the vast majority were determined by one's high school exams and a subsequent "standard assessment test" for medical students. The exam tested forms of intelligence that were supposedly important for studying medicine, such as logical thinking, spatial reasoning, and mathematical ability. Despite spending 450 Deutschmarks on a preparation course taught by an enterprising psychologist, I didn't do exceptionally well on that test, either. I was counting on a long waiting period, and now I had received this invitation for a selection interview. Finally, on March 17, 1989—I still remember it as though it were yesterday; it was a Friday and Marc Almond and Gene Pitney were on top of the charts with "Something's Gotten Hold of My Heart"—I received my acceptance into the medical program at the Freie Universität zu Berlin.

What Happened with Susanne Sieckler?

I began this book with her story; I would like to finish with it as well. Susanne listened as Dr. Fernandez-Meier, who was substituting for her colleague, told her the bad news that her cancer had grown despite the chemotherapy. She received the announcement calmly, quickly forgetting about her long wait for the doctor, and then managed to arrive in time for the lantern festival at her daughter's school. That had been her real goal this afternoon—not the results, not a new treatment plan, just the lantern festival.

The parade wound its way through the streets of Susanne's childhood, past the former apartment of the beloved German children's author Erich Kästner, up to the famous Prager Platz. It was wonderful—as she and her daughter sang, there was no illness, no bad results, and no bad news—just the wonderful feeling of being a live. "My daughter was so proud of the lantern that we made together—a pink papier-mâché dragon. It was one of the loveliest experiences in my life to that point," she told me when we met several months later.

Currently, Ms. Sieckler is receiving treatment as part of a study on "maintenance therapy" and is responding very well. The tumor has stopped growing, she reports to me in the outpatient clinic. Just as we are about to say goodbye, her doctor passes by. Her real doctor, the one she trusts the most and who has cared for her for months, the same doctor who had to tell Susanne the most difficult news of her life: Dr. Fernandez-Meier.

Appendix: Help for Helpers, Recipients, and Relatives

CONTENTS

Brief Summary of the SPIKES Method

(See Baile et al., 2000 in Bibliography)

1. *S—Setting up the interview*: Preparation, general situation, physical settings, prevent and/or minimize interruptions, involve significant others.

2. *P—Assessing the patient's perception*: Receptivity + Level of information and awareness, determining the patient's expectations, "before you tell—ask."

3. *I—Obtaining the patient's invitation*: How open is the patient to receiving information? Don't disregard the patient's right to *not* know (consult first), which of their close friends or relatives should be present at the conversation?

4. *K—Giving knowledge and information to the patient*: Determine the goal of the conversation before communicating bad news; always begin with a warning before finally communicating the "bad" news. Use simple sentences, don't overload the conversation with too much information, pause and wait after delivering important information or statements, and make sure the recipient has understood the important information.

5. *E—Addressing the patient's emotions*: Listen, observe the situation and the patient's reaction, stay receptive to and respectful of the patient's emotions, show empathy.

6. *S—Providing strategy and summary*: Try and involve patients in active decision making regarding next steps; let them participate. A brief summary of the conversation and discussing subsequent steps at the end can help orient patients. Next steps might include potential medical measures such as beginning treatment for pain, referral to another doctor, organizing home care, or setting an appointment for a follow-up conversation.

Guidelines for Announcing a Death

Adapted from F. Lasogga and B. Gasch (*Notfallpsychologie*, 2004)

What Do I Do before Announcing a Death?

- Before giving news of the death, gather as much information about the deceased and his or her relatives and/or life partner as possible (quality of relationship, profession, current circumstances).
- Don't communicate the tragic news by phone (setting up a meeting in person is possible, however).
- Plan on anywhere from 15 to 45 minutes, and think about who might stay with the relatives and/or life partner of the deceased after (i.e., potentially bring in pastoral care or professional help).
- Expect—and respect—a wide range of reactions and emotions: anger, crying, bewilderment, despair, apathy, shock, and aggression.
- Include and/or alert professional help ahead of time (pastoral care, crisis specialists, emergency doctors), or invite them in after the initial conversation.

What Do I Do When It Is Time?

- Make sure you are speaking about the right person.
- The person communicating the news should introduce himself or herself and the institution he or she works for by name, and state his or her position (e.g., police, paramedic, hospital attendant, or social worker).
- Warn the recipient ahead of time of the impending bad news. Pause briefly before continuing.
- Ask the recipient whom they would like to stay with them or to come.
- Maintain eye contact; try to project a sense of stability and calm through your body language.
- As far as possible, try to determine the immediate recipient's relationship to any other people present.
- Speak clearly, slowly, and understandably about what has happened, avoiding professional terminology if at all possible.
- Speak clearly about "death" or "dead" rather than talking around the subject. At the same time, don't refer to "the deceased," but rather "your wife," "your husband," or "your child."
- Answer any questions honestly and truthfully.
- Listen actively to the recipient, taking the recipient's reactions fully into consideration. Refrain from speaking too much once you have delivered the necessary information, allow for silence and don't interrupt with cliché phrases, as well-intentioned as these may be.
- Try not to leave the recipient alone, that is, help him or her to contact people or take the next immediate steps.

- Leave the recipient with a list of addresses that relatives, friends, or anyone else who has been affected can contact for help (pastoral care, self-help groups, emergency psychologists, etc.).

Breaking Bad News: Seminars

Seminars provide doctors with an ideal opportunity to reflect and improve on their communication skills. In principle, various positions within the healthcare system such as nurses and doctor's assistants, but also other fields such as police or paramedics concepts also stand to benefit greatly from engaging in these topics.

We try to limit the number of participants in our seminars to between 12 and 15 people, in order to encourage intimate and intensive conversation.

Together with my colleague Dr. Christine Klapp, I've conducted intensive seminars of this sort for nearly 20 years. Participants come from a wide range of disciplines: gynecologists, internal medicine specialists, anesthesiologists, urologists, and emergency medical personnel.

When assembling a list of participants, it is important to watch for any potential conflicts in hierarchy within the group. I clearly remember one seminar in which one assistant began crying after a head doctor criticized her heavily during a feedback session, faulting her for a lack of professional experience. He did so despite the fact that the assistant's conversational techniques were much more comfortable and better suited to the simulation patient than were those of the head doctor. I notice again and again how a strict, hierarchically structured medical system with specialists, assistant directors, and head physicians limits a group's ability for dialogue. Although horizontal structures encourage discussion, they are by no means a precondition for constructive criticism, or the all-important culture of conversation.

During seminars, it is participants' attitude and ability to take criticism that matter the most. Practicing constructive criticism and receiving criticism, even when it is not constructive: those are virtues that doctors—and not only doctors—have not necessarily been taught. In their everyday hospital work, doctors are often faced only with extreme forms of feedback. A bouquet or box of chocolates on the one hand, on the other a written complaint sent directly to the medical director, or a letter from a lawyer making a formal accusation of medical malpractice. Especially when it comes to negative criticism, much is written, but little spoken: conversations are rare. Giving and receiving criticism are learnable, however.

One precondition for fostering a good conversational atmosphere is allowing participants to absorb conversations intellectually and emotionally without needing to immediately assess their value. This type of observation is not only directed at others' conversations and reflections, but also at one's own, and provides a sort of external view of oneself.

We try to design the seminars to be as practical as possible and to allow room for "actively stepping back" and discussion. For most participants, it is the first time in their professional career they have attended a workshop of this kind, and it takes time until they begin to reflect consciously on doctor–patient conversations and to share experiences with their colleagues.

Again and again during these courses, we find that articulating personal experiences in a professional environment (i.e., among one's colleagues) is uncharted territory for many.

The seminar can be designed to last different amounts of time depending on the concept and goals, ranging from 2 days up to a full curriculum that takes several months to complete, and includes various exercises such as role-play scenarios and simulation patients.

Setting out the course program in advance helps participants to continually reengage at the professional, factual level. Short, pointed presentations on the theoretical background of the course material further help participants approach the topic intellectually as well as emotionally.

The various exercises we use in our seminars are based on everyday experiences in the hospital; participants are also invited to share their own experiences and patient histories.

By means of role-plays and the use of "simulation patients," these stories are then brought back into the present and acted out in real time.

Such role-play scenarios make participants aware of different perspectives, often reminding them of difficult, long-forgotten conversations they have had over the course of their own career.

In their feedback, seminar participants regularly mention that it is the first time in their professional lives they have taken time to reflect on their patterns of communication. Many view it as a "true luxury" to be able to engage with the subject.

Because participants usually have not undergone any training as actors, they do not always "stick to the script" of the role-play or their task descriptions. Now and then, emotionally difficult situations may be met with comedy, humor, or foolishness, with participants breaking out of their role and bringing an early end to the intended conversation. Many participants may also have insufficient practice expressing criticism.

Role-plays help participants to develop observation skills. Simulation patients are far and away the best method for practicing communication. We adapt the different roles to the specific group of participants and try to fully explore a situation, for example, delivering the initial diagnosis for a severe medical case (e.g., fatal accident, breast cancer, HIV, ovarian cancer), an incurable recurrence, or situations in which no other forms of treatment are possible and it must be assumed that the patient will die soon.

Simulation patients are trained actors that bring a predetermined medical history with them, featuring an extensive résumé that includes professional and personal relationships and situations. They behave authentically and react during the conversations in such a way as to have the greatest training effect possible on participants.

Following the conversation, which plays out before the entire group, the simulation patient leaves the room and switches hats, so to speak. He or she then returns to the group to give feedback to the person who communicated the news.

First, the person sharing the bad news is asked how they felt during the conversation— what in their opinion went well, and what didn't go as well. As a final question, the person can be asked whether he or she thinks that he or she effectively communicated whatever information had to be passed on, and how he or she imagines the patient felt at the end of the conversation—whether anything may have been left unsaid that he or she might have liked to ask the patient.

The simulation patient is then asked the same questions. They have been specially trained to formulate their critiques and always look to highlight positive aspects and improve trainees' confidence. Participants report again and again how quickly they find themselves immersed in the situation, completely forgetting about the artificial parameters and perceiving it as real. I regularly see tears in the eyes of participants who are only observing.

When holding conversations with simulation patients, it is possible at any moment to start over again with different phrases or information, repeating the situation in order to guide the discussion in another direction. I myself thought this was possible only in training seminars until several months ago. I was speaking with a patient at the hospital and could feel that something wasn't right about our chemistry—I told her as much and asked her if we could start the conversation over again. "I feel as though I haven't guided you through this conversation about your difficult medical situation very well. Would it be alright with you if we took a short break and began again?" She listened quietly although I could also feel her anger, then she looked up and said, "By all means; I'm also thirsty." I brought her a green tea, and we started the conversation over again. We spoke for about a half an hour, and at the end I had a good feeling despite having to communicate very serious medical findings. The patient also thanked me later for the second and, in her mind as well, better try. I recommend not entirely discounting this option and trying it as a plan B when needed.

Various studies indicate that over the long term, doctors who have gone through similar training courses handle difficult conversations more effectively, and themselves experience lower levels of stress. At the same time, it should be stated that to date only a small number of studies have been conducted on these effects over the long term, and most did not involve the affected patients.

Even without proof in the sense of "evidence-based medicine," in my view, it is still important that such forms of training are required not only during medical study but also in specialist training, and after. Without regular fine-tuning, we fall back into old patterns all too quickly. This is the case with nearly every medical technique or procedure. Engaging in a structured, concrete (and guided) manner with how to communicate bad news can also positively impact the motivation that doctors and medical staff alike feel for practicing their profession, another result studies have clearly shown. Well-timed, regular "stops" of this sort can also reduce the risk of burnout among medical personnel.

Checklists for Communicating Bad News

For the Bearer

1. Have I spent enough time preparing?

   When do we meet? Time constraints? What are my own motivations? Do I know what the recipient knows already (current physical, psychological, social, and emotional situation)? Is the recipient prepared for what I have to say? What might be next steps after the conversation?

2. How do I gather any necessary information about my counterpart during the conversation?

   What signals is the recipient communicating, verbally and nonverbally?

   What does the recipient know? What does he want to know? Can I determine his level of information?

3. How and when do I warn my counterpart?

   Give a warning early on that bad news will soon follow. The sooner the better.

4. Use pauses and open questions, avoid interrupting.

   Using pauses and open questions gives recipients a chance to process the bad news and to express their own thoughts and emotions.

5. Stay focused on the essential message of the bad news.

   Avoid using sentences that are too long. Allow the essential message to have its effect without relativizing or glossing it over, or switching to other topics. Use the power of the pause.

6. Make repeated offers for practical and pragmatic help.

7. Sum up the conversation, emphasizing "the positive side" whenever possible. Name potential next steps.

   Don't force your search for the "positive side." What is good from your point of view as the one giving the news may be "bad" from the recipient's point of view.

8. Debriefing.

   Unwind after the conversation by speaking with someone or taking a short break before going back to work.

For Recipients

This list can also be used to help prepare the person sharing the bad news. Incorporating the perspective of the recipient and his relatives is always helpful.

1. How can I prepare for the conversation?

   Can I help set a time? Do I want to have somebody I trust with me? Who should be there if it is good news? If it is bad news?

2. How can I best absorb all the information I hear?

   Ask follow-up questions or request that your companion take notes. As a general rule, however, conversations with bad news often contain too much, not too little information. You can find out more information later, in subsequent conversations.

3. Ask for pauses, try to express your own emotions and thoughts.

   Take all the time you need to orient yourself and continue following the conversation. If it is simply too much, say so, and ask for a break.

4. Focus on the essential message of the bad news.

   What is the key message? Have I understood it? Can I describe it to my loved ones?

5. Ask the person communicating the bad news to summarize the conversation at the end. How can I best be helped now?

   What might the next practical steps be? Who can support me? Who can accompany me through the grief and uncertainty? Who can I stay with today? How do I get home? What has helped me before in dealing with bad news?

For Companions

1. How can I prepare for the conversation?

   What do I know about the previous course the illness and conversations have taken? How serious is the situation now? Am I willing and able to cope with the situation? Does the affected person want me to be present?

2. Observe the conversation.

   How can I best grasp all the information delivered during the conversation? What roles can and should I take on? Ask the person who is directly impacted.

3. Bear with the situation.

   The rhythm of the conversation should be dictated only by the recipient and bearer of the bad news. Don't try and play the role of moderator or lawyer, but rather be present as a silent observer—one who can ask questions, of course.

4. Focus on the essential message of the bad news.

   What is the essential message? Have I understood it?

5. After the conversation.

   Once it is over, offer to discuss the conversation and summary again. If, however, the person no longer wishes to talk about it for the moment, this should also be respected. Try to focus on providing practical assistance, such as organizing a ride home or shopping. Ask the person if you should stay with him or her, and offer to listen to them. Don't pressure yourself to immediately come up with perfect solutions.

6. Self-reflection.

   How do I best reflect on my role and effect in handling the bad news? Who can help me deal with the emotions and thoughts of being an "extra burden?" Do I need professional support?

Bibliography of Selected Scientific Research

Aizer AA, Chen MH, McCarthy EP et al. Marital status and survival in patients with cancer. *J Clin Oncol*. 2013;31(31):3869–3876.

Baile WF, Buckman R, Lenzi R et al. SPIKES—A six-step protocol for delivering bad news: Application to the patient with cancer. *Oncologist*. 2000;5:302–311.

Diehm, M. *Sehouli: Mit Schreiben zur Lebenskraft*. Übungsbuch für Frauen mit Krebserkrankungen und ihre Angehöigen, München, 2018.

Fallowfield LJ, Jenkins V, Farewell V, Saul J, Duffy A, Eves R. Efficacy of a Cancer Research UK communication skills training model for oncologists: A randomized controlled trial. *Lancet*. 2011;359:650–656.

Harvard School of Public Health. *The Burden of Stress in America*. National Public Radio (U.S.). Princeton, NJ: Robert Wood Johnson Foundation; 2014.

Holman EA, Fargin Dr, Silver RC. Media's role in broadcasting acute stress following the Boston Marathon bombings. 2014;111(1):93–98. doi: 10.1073/pnas.1316265110

Klapp C. Kommunikation—praktische Tipps fur das schwierige Gespräch mit Patienten. *Gynakol Geburtsmed Gynakol Endokrinol*. 2010;6(2):152–166.

Oskay-Özcelik G, Lehmacher W, Könsgen D et al. Breast cancer patients' expectations in respect of the physician-patient relationship and treatment management results of a survey of 617 patients. *Ann Oncol.* 2007;18:479–484.

Romer G, Bergelt C, Möller B. *Kinder krebskranker Eltern: Manual zur kindzentrierten Familiesnberatung nach dem COSIP-Konzept.* Hogrefe Verlag; Auflage: 1 (June 11, 2014).

Vorderwülbecke F, Feistle M, Mehring M, Schneider A, Linde K. Aggression and violence against primary care physicians, a nationwide questionnaire survey. *Dtsch Arztebl Int* 2015;112:159.

Index

A

Anamnesis, 4, 5

B

Bad news, 1, 58; *see also* Breaking bad
   news
  assimilating, 38–44
  coping mechanisms, 38
  and decisive question, 28–30
  difficulties in understanding, 25–26
  doctor–patient conversation, 16–20
  final goals of patient, 43
  informational gap, 31–32
  learning from life experience,
    44–45
  obsessing over negative news,
    58–59
  overcoming, 12–14
  and patient's reaction, 41–42
  and stress, 58
Bad news communication checklist, 75
  for bearer, 75–76
  for companions, 77
  for recipients, 76
Balint group, 49
Breaking bad news, 11
  art of, 67
  art of *not* speaking, 26–28
  being aware of one's role, 21–24
  being sympathetic, 22–23
  conversation documentation, 48–49
  conversation initiation, 24
  conversing with children, 49–51
  doctor–patient communications,
    2–3
  doctor's perspective, 3
  emotion and vulnerability in, 9–10
  employee termination, 54–55

familiarizing with lay concepts,
    32–35
head doctor's visit, 11–12
learning to, 2, 5–9
in mythology, 1–2
police, 51–53
preparing for existential
    conversation, 14–16
responsibility of, 4–5
role-play scenarios, 74
seminars, 73–75
simulated conversation, 39–40
simulation patients, 39, 74–75
social dimension of health, 16
SPIKES system, 15–16
spirituality, 46–48
training for, 7
truthfulness and trust, 30–32
turning relatives into allies, 35–38

C

Cancer, endometrial, 4
Child-centered family counseling, 51
Children of Somatically Ill Parents
    (COSIP), 51
Clinical study as alternative treatment
    form, 33
Computed tomography (CT), 12, 58
Conversational protocol, 48
Coping mechanisms, 38; *see also*
    Breaking bad news
  final goals of patient, 43
  physical reactions from patients,
    41–42
  resilience, 38–39
  simulated conversation, 39–40
  writing, 44
Cortisone treatment, 23

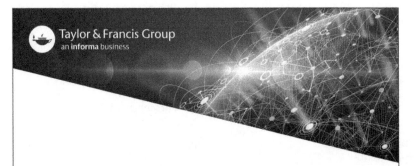